PMS

PREMENSTRUAL
SYNDROME

PMS

Premenstrual Syndrome

A Guide for Young Women

Gilda Berger

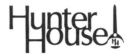

Third edition ©1991 by Gilda Berger

Originally published under the title *PMS: Premenstrual Syndrome* by Franklin Watts, 1984

Photograph opposite page 1 courtesy of Conklin from Monkmeyer Press Photo Service
Grateful acknowledgment is given for permission to reprint copyrighted illustrations on p. 10 from *Once A Month* by Katharina Dalton, M.D., published by Hunter House Inc., Publishers

Hunter House, Inc.
2200 Central Ave., Suite 202
Alameda, CA 94501-4451

Library of Congress Cataloging in Publication Data:

Berger, Gilda.
    PMS, premenstrual syndrome : a guide for young women / Gilda Berger. — 3rd ed.
    p. cm.
    Includes bibliographical references and index.
    Summary: Discusses the symptoms, causes, and treatment of premenstrual syndrome, or PMS
    ISBN 0-89793-088-6 : $7.95
    1. Premenstrual syndrome—Juvenile literature.
[1. Premenstrual syndrome.] I. Title
RG165.B47   1991
618.1'72—dc20   91-34647
                                     CIP
                                     AC

Editorial Coordinator: Lisa E. Lee
Production Manager: Paul J. Frindt
Publisher: Kiran S. Rana
Cover design: Ellen Perry and Qalagraphia.
Text set in 11 on 13 point Palatino; titles in Avant Garde
Manufactured in the United States of America

9 8 7 6 5 4 3 2 1   Third edition

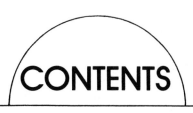

CONTENTS

CHAPTER 1
"The World's Commonest Disease"
1

CHAPTER 2
The Menstrual Cycle
7

CHAPTER 3
The Physical Symptoms of PMS
17

CHAPTER 4
The Psychological Symptoms of PMS
27

CHAPTER 5
Causes of PMS
35

CHAPTER 6
Self-Help for PMS
45

CHAPTER 7
Going to the Doctor for PMS
59

CHAPTER 8
Social and Legal Issues
69

Bibliography
79

Appendix
81

Index
83

FOR HEIDI B.

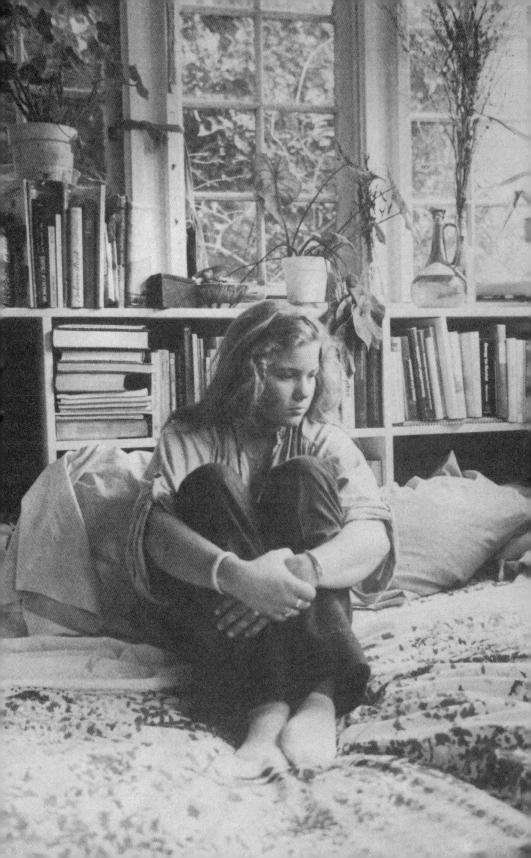

1

"THE WORLD'S COMMONEST DISEASE."

Sally W. of New Haven, Connecticut, used to feel she was not one, but two different people. "From the time I was sixteen, I was a real Jekyll and Hyde," she has often said.

For three weeks of every month Sally felt normal, intelligent, attractive, and well-adjusted. But the week before her menstrual period, she became irritable, depressed, clumsy, and completely out of control. She suffered with painful headaches, cried for no reason, became forgetful, and picked fights with everyone.

Over the years, Sally went to a number of doctors seeking help. They offered remedies to relieve her tension and anxiety, treat her irritability, and cure the headaches, backaches, and even the weight gain that troubled her at this particular time of every month. Some of the treatments helped a little; many made her feel even worse.

What was most discouraging was that none of the doctors really seemed to understand what was wrong. Sally's complaints kept intensifying. She began to fear that she was going insane, and worried that one day she would end up in a mental hospital.

A few of Sally's friends and her parents convinced her that her troubles were probably "all in her head." So she sought the help of a psychiatrist. It was this therapist who told her that she was not going mad, but probably suffering from a very common disorder, called PMS, or premenstrual syndrome. (*Pre* means before; *menstrual* refers to the monthly cycle of the female reproductive system; and *syndrome* is a group of symptoms that appear together.) Dr. Katharina Dalton, one of the world's leading experts on PMS, defines it simply as the "symptoms or complaints which regularly come just before or during menstruation but are absent at other times of the cycle." While millions of women have endured PMS for centuries, it is just now being recognized as a specific condition, and is being studied and written about.

Sally's doctor explained the monthly changes occurring within her body that caused the physical, psychological, and emotional symptoms of PMS, and gave her much useful information on how to lessen or eliminate the symptoms. Just learning that she was not alone, and not mentally ill, made Sally feel better than she had felt in years. Sally made up her mind to gain control over her body. With some changes in diet and exercise, Sally began to feel like herself—not just some of the time—but always.

PMS: WHAT IS IT?

PMS is a medical problem characterized by a group of symptoms that appears one to fourteen days before menstruation and disappears once menstruation actually starts. Doctors list about 150 possible physical and psychological symptoms. No one ever gets all of them at once; most sufferers, though, have several symptoms and in varying degrees of severity.

The most common symptoms, according to Dr. Ronald V. Norris, who set up the first American clinic for PMS in 1981, are tension and irritability; bloating; swelling of the ankles, feet, or fingers; weight gain; and headaches. Other frequently reported complaints include fatigue and depression, crying for no reason, backaches, pimples or other skin disorders, a craving for sweets, and clumsiness.

Of course, these symptoms also appear in people who do not have PMS. But the difference is that in women with PMS, the symptoms show up in relation to the menstrual cycle. If no menstrual pattern is present, these women probably do not have PMS.

Medical students are now being taught the connection between PMS and the "Three Ps." PMS can occur after a girl reaches *puberty*, or sexual maturity. Sometimes it starts after a woman's first *pregnancy*. And stopping the use of the birth control *pill* can cause the symptoms to either start or become more severe.

In general, PMS is believed to worsen with age and childbearing. For many women, the distress increases and the symptoms grow more severe until menopause, around age fifty, when menstruation ceases.

Almost all women in their childbearing years, an estimated 85 percent, says Dr. Norris, experience PMS occasionally. About 40 percent have PMS regularly. And between 10 and 15 percent endure pain and discomfort severe enough to disrupt their lives. Is it any wonder that Dr. Dalton calls it "the world's commonest disease"?

PMS: WHAT IT IS NOT

PMS is *not* menstrual cramps or the pain that may occur during menstruation. In fact, for most women with PMS, the menstrual period offers relief from their symptoms. As one doctor put it, PMS victims "look forward to bleeding."

PMS and menstrual cramps are not related. The pain that comes with menstruation has a different cause than the difficulties associated with PMS. The way to tell them apart is to watch when they occur. Those associated with menstruation start at the time of your period, last two or three days, and disappear. The symptoms of PMS appear *before* the start of your period and disappear soon after its onset.

PMS is also *not* a psychological problem. It was once thought, for example, that PMS was a kind of depression found only among women. But leading researchers have found otherwise. Dr. Roger Haskell, a psychiatrist at the University of Michigan, has found that PMS sufferers show none of the common signs of serious depression. Dr. Dalton and others who have treated thousands of women with PMS have found that once the medical problems of the condition are cleared up, the depression and other psychological problems ease or go away altogether.

You may have had the symptoms of PMS since puberty. Perhaps your mother, older sister, or other close relative has suffered the same complaints, too. Still, that is no reason for you to continue to put up with PMS month after month. PMS is not a natural part of growing up female. There are now ways to get relief from the disturbances of PMS.

THE PROBLEM

PMS was not recognized as a medical condition until 1931, when Dr. Robert T. Frank wrote an article in a medical journal describing the disorder. Why did it take the medical profession so long to take notice of PMS?

One possible reason is that women used to have larger families. While they were pregnant or breast-feeding they were free of menstruation. Modern women tend to have far fewer children. Therefore, the probability of PMS symptoms showing up in women today is greatly increased.

Since primitive times, too, women have been taught that they were supposed to suffer through the menstrual cycle each month. When they complained, they were told, "It's all in your head," or "Just learn to live with it," or "Quit the complaining."

The old belief that menstruation was a punishment wrought by God on women probably sprang from the story of Adam and Eve. According to the Book of Genesis in the Bible, a serpent in the Garden of Eden tempted Eve to eat the forbidden fruit of the tree of knowledge, and she led Adam to eat also. For this disobedience they were both punished. Until recently, menstruation was called "the curse," and the pain, discomfort, and depression commonly associated with it were considered part of women's penance for Eve's transgression.

No one knows how much the attitudes of society act upon PMS. But almost everyone believes that they do have some effect. The plain fact is that the less you understand and respect your body, the less able you are to deal with the changes that do take place.

Traditionally, most doctors have been male. For years women have taken their complaints to them and been told that there was no physical basis for the fatigue, aches and pains, nervousness, and other common symptoms of PMS. The monthly difficulties were either ignored, misdiagnosed, or erroneously treated. Perhaps it is not surprising, then, that the first advance in PMS research, after Dr. Frank, was made by a woman, Dr. Katharina Dalton, in the early 1950s.

THE REMEDY

Dr. Dalton became aware of PMS after she noticed that she had a migraine headache just before the onset of every menses, or period. She also found that a patient whom she was treating for repeated attacks of asthma suffered these attacks at the same time every month. Then two more patients came along—one with headaches, the other with asthma. They both showed the same cyclical pattern of symptoms preceding menstruation.

After interviewing eighty-seven other women who also suffered some form of distress before the onset of their menses, Dr. Dalton published her findings in a number of medical journals and books. She attracted notice at once and became the leading authority in investigating and developing methods for treating the condition. By now, Dr. Dalton has treated over 22,000 patients in the PMS clinic at University College Hospital in London, England. Her work has inspired many others.

PMS specialists and researchers are now at work on this disorder in countries around the world. Emphasizing the importance of diet, stress reduction, exercise, vitamin therapy, and the use of a female sex hormone—progesterone, they have helped many women and their families to improve their life situations.

Still, despite the many advances, much remains to be done. PMS is an extremely complex condition. It is also a peculiar malady, with symptoms varying from individual to individual. Just as the causes may differ, so do the treatments. All therapies succeed sometimes; none work all the time. But with the help now available, and new understanding growing rapidly, many women with PMS can be helped.

2

THE MENSTRUAL CYCLE

Puberty, which occurs at any time from age eight to thirteen, but usually around eleven, is a very important event in every girl's life. It is followed by the first menstruation, called the menarche, about two years later.

Menstruation is the once-a-month discharge of blood that lasts approximately three to five days. It is the end result of an ongoing series of complex hormonal and anatomical changes that occur in a woman's body in preparation for a possible pregnancy. From the menarche on, menstruation is part of every woman's biorhythm for the next thirty years or so. The only time it does not occur is during pregnancy. The end of menstruation, known as menopause, takes place at about age fifty.

To understand premenstrual syndrome, you need to know about the menstrual cycle and the many individual body changes that take place from one menstrual period to the next.

MENSTRUATION:
STEP BY STEP

The normal monthly sequence of events that ends in menstruation is known as the menstrual cycle. The cycle begins the day the bleeding starts. The hypothalamus, a walnut-shaped unit of the brain, sends out tiny spurts of chemical messengers known as hormones. From the hypothalamus, the hormones travel to the pituitary gland, which is also in the brain. They stimulate the pituitary to produce its own hormones.

The first hormone from the pituitary gland is known as FSH (Follicle Stimulating Hormone). The hormone is carried by the bloodstream to the two female sex glands, the ovaries. Each ovary—oval in shape, about one and one-half inches long, and pinkish gray in color—contains a lifetime supply of up to 500,000 unripe egg cells. FSH causes one of the eggs to begin ripening within a tiny sac, known as a follicle. Usually only one egg matures during each menstrual cycle. (Eggs that have not been used disintegrate at menopause.)

The ovaries' follicles also produce hormones. One of these is a sex hormone called estrogen. Estrogen, among other functions, leads the glands that line the uterus, or womb, to form a new lining (the endometrium). This prepares the uterus to receive the egg, should it meet and become united with a sperm through sexual intercourse.

About ten to fourteen days after the beginning of menstruation, the egg cell is mature. It looks a little like a puffy blister on the inner surface of the ovary. The pituitary now releases another hormone, LH (Luteinizing Hormone). This makes the ovary release the mature egg, a step known as ovulation. The span of time from the beginning of menstruation until ovulation is referred to as the follicular phase of the menstrual cycle.

The released egg now passes slowly (it takes about three to five days) from the ovary through the fallopian tubes to the uterus. The fallopian tubes are narrow passageways that connect the ovaries to the uterus. While the egg is traveling to the uterus, the LH is bringing about changes in the empty follicle which held the egg. The broken-down follicle turns yellow (it is called corpus luteum or yellow body), and begins to produce two sex hormones, progesterone and estrogen. The progesterone helps to build up the endometrium and makes it soft and spongy.

If a woman has sexual intercourse shortly after ovulation, fertilization may take place in the fallopian tube. This joining of the egg and sperm is called conception. The fertilized egg then attaches to the lining of the uterus, thick and spongy with blood vessels and fluids. The lining nourishes the fertilized egg. With fertilization, the menstrual cycle stops until after the birth of the baby.

Most often, though, the egg does not become fertilized. Therefore, it does not attach itself to the uterine lining. Instead, the egg dies after a day or so. The pituitary, reacting to the high level of estrogen and progesterone produced by the corpus luteum in the ovary, now lowers its production of LH. The drop in LH causes the corpus luteum to decay, and the levels of progesterone and estrogen drop, too.

When these hormone levels reach a certain low point, the lining in the uterus begins to break down and fall off. This falling off, or shedding, causes the bleeding that we call menstruation, menstrual period, or menses. The bleeding washes most of the lining of the uterus out of your body. It marks the completion of one complete menstrual cycle. This second phase of the cycle, from ovulation to the onset of menses, takes approximately fourteen days, and is known as the luteal phase.

A day or two later, the hypothalamus, sensing the absence of estrogen and progesterone in the blood,

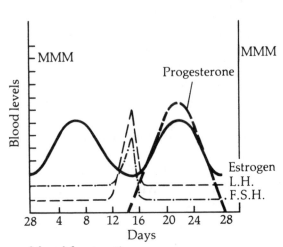

Female hormone levels during the
menstrual cycle

M = Menstruation

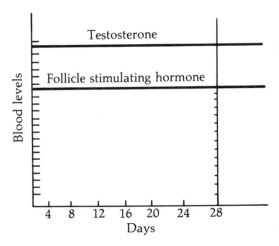

Male hormone levels during a month

sends neurotransmitters to the pituitary gland. The new
menstrual cycle is under way.

MENSTRUAL
DIFFICULTIES

The menstrual cycle, as you can probably imagine, is
extremely delicate. The wonder is not that things can go
wrong. The marvel is that it works at all!

Problems often arise that may make regular menstrual periods irregular in some way. These problems
should not be confused with PMS, which presents itself
before the onset of the menses.

Often, young women may skip their menstrual
period for two months or more. Some may bleed on and
off between periods, experience excessive bleeding during the period itself, or, what is more common, have
menstrual cramps or pain during menstruation.

What causes such irregularities? Sometimes late
and heavy bleeding problems arise because you are
menstruating but not yet ovulating. That is, you're not
producing an egg and not having a monthly rise and fall
of hormones. Your ovaries, though, are producing
estrogen irregularly without producing the progesterone
needed to control the uterine lining buildup.

Heavy bleeding may be the result of excessive
development of the uterine lining and blood vessels.
Bleeding may begin, for example, six or seven weeks
after your last period. The bleeding may be heavy and
last longer. Sometimes persistent disruption in hormonal patterns can result in a starting-and-stopping pattern.
For example, you may bleed for five days, stop for five
days, bleed for seven, stop for twelve, and so on.

Doctors sometimes try to correct ovulation and hor-
monal-balance problems with medication, usually natural progesterone or artificial progesterone.

Stress and fatigue may affect the menstrual cycle.

To study their impact on menstruation, Dr. Dalton conducted a study in England that involved 100 high school girls. Normally sixteen girls out of the sample were menstruating on any particular day. During the week of final exams in June, though, Dr. Dalton found that the number shot up to thirty-six!

Stress is believed to cause a lack of adjustment between the hypothalamus and the pituitary gland. When you are tense and upset, these two areas of the brain may interfere with each other. The interference results in fluctuation of the sex hormones, leading to irregular menstruation.

One young woman began to bleed after she learned both of her parents had been killed in a car accident, even though she was not at that point in her cycle. What probably happened was that her hypothalamus became inactive because of the shock. There was a sudden drop in stimulation of the ovaries. The ovaries stopped producing estrogen, and that produced the bleeding.

If you are over seventeen and under forty-five and not pregnant, and are not having menstrual periods (amenorrhea), there may be a problem with the hormone release from the brain. Sometimes the pituitary gland is not stimulated. The ovaries, in turn, do not release normal amounts of estrogen and progesterone. Amenorrhea due to the suppression of hormones from the hypothalamus may result from illness, travel, a sudden drop in weight, or stress caused by the breakup of a romance, entering college, or starting a new job, for example.

Almost every woman has menstrual cramps at one time or another at the onset of the menses. It is a common problem that is not very well understood. Severe menstrual cramps without any underlying medical problem are most common among teenagers. The difficulty, also called spasmodic dysmenorrhea, often appears in the first year or so after periods begin. In addition to a mild cramping pain on one side or another of the abdomen, you may feel pain in the upper parts of your thighs and the lower back. Nausea, vomiting, diarrhea, headaches, and lack of appetite may also accompany the cramps and pain. Spasmodic dysmenorrhea rarely lasts more than two or three days within each cycle, and usually lessens after age twenty-five. Childbirth, too, almost always puts an end to menstrual cramps.

A very common problem, dysmenorrhea is responsible for an estimated 140 million lost working hours each year in the United States alone. Although no one knows the exact cause of menstrual cramps, the problem is now believed to be caused by high levels of prostaglandins, hormones that stimulate contractions in the uterus. The higher the concentration of prostaglandins at the time of menstruation, the stronger and more frequent the uterine contractions. Women with low prostaglandin production may have little or no menstrual pain. For this reason, some doctors now use antiprostaglandins in the treatment of dysmenorrhea.

Dr. Dalton and some others feel that the immediate cause of the pain is the uterine muscle contracting in an attempt to shed the uterine lining. Very strong contractions over a long time can decrease blood flow to the muscle causing pain. Also, the flow of blood, they believe, puts a strain on the neck of the uterus.

As you get older the pain lessens. That is because the uterus gains better control over the menstrual flow. Childbearing seems to lessen cramps because the mouth of the womb becomes enlarged, permitting easier passage of the menstrual material. If the cramps are severe, you may want to see a doctor. If no serious medical problem is present, you may try some self-help techniques that have helped others.

To our primitive ancestors, menstruation must have been a very frightening and bewildering occurrence. Many myths developed around this completely natural event. Some of these strange ideas persist even today, and may affect the way you deal with menstruation.

You may suffer under the ancient notion, for example, that menstruation is somehow "bad." You may have grown up with negative attitudes you acquired from your parents or friends. Perhaps you were taught to hide all evidence of menstruation. It may be that you were mistakenly told to avoid baths or shampoos when you are menstruating, or warned that a cold shower could reduce the menstrual flow. No one really knows how much poor attitudes can affect menstrual discomfort, but false, negative beliefs can cause stress and anxiety and disturb normal functioning. One girl brought up in a very religious home says, "I still want to run and hide when I get my period."

If you have spasmodic dysmenorrhea, with no underlying medical illness, you can benefit from simple relaxation and breathing exercises. In one experiment, Dr. Dalton separated a number of college students with spasmodic dysmenorrhea into three groups. One group received relaxation exercises five times a week. Another was given psychological counseling. And the third was left untreated. Later, all the students were questioned on the effect of the treatment on their pain. Only those who did the relaxation exercises reported dramatic and long-ranging relief and improvement of their condition.

Most people agree that heat helps to relax cramped, tight muscles in the pelvis and lower back, and for relieving aches in the legs. Taking a warm bath or resting with a heating pad on your lower abdomen for about thirty minutes, will often make you feel better.

Occasionally, relief can come from aspirin or similar over-the-counter compounds sold in drug stores. For the best results, you should take these pain killers at the very first sign of discomfort.

In general, any steps you take to improve your overall health and condition will also lessen the pain or discomfort of irregular menstruation. Suggested guidelines are: plan a daily exercise program; eat a varied, well-balanced diet; get plenty of rest; and make every effort to reduce unnecessary stress and tension. Research indicates that such a regime will surely help.

3

THE PHYSICAL SYMPTOMS OF PMS

In the week or so before your period:
>Do you have splitting headaches?
>Do parts of your body swell, making
>   you feel as heavy as an elephant?
>Do your breasts feel tender?
>Do things fall out of your hands, and
>   do you feel clumsier than usual?
>Does your face break out?

When your period begins:
>Do your headaches disappear?
>Do the swellings go down?
>Do your breasts feel normal?
>Are you as well-coordinated as usual?
>Does your complexion clear up?

If you said yes to some or all of the above questions, you may have the physical symptoms of PMS. Until recently, the annoying, sometimes painful, signs of this disorder went unreported and unrecognized.

Now, because PMS is recognized as a very real medical problem and its symptoms have been identified, the situation is much different. You can decide if you have these or other complaints. You can find out whether or not they follow a regular pattern. And, if you discover that you do have the physical symptoms of PMS, you can take steps to bring them under control.

HEADACHES

Headaches are often called the body's all-purpose distress signal. They alert you to the fact that something is wrong. Although they have many origins, we do know that headaches occur more often in women than in men. Many seem to be clearly related to the menstrual cycle.

One study of boys and girls shows a similar incidence in the severe migraine-type of headache between the ages of seven and thirteen. After age thirteen, however, when most girls had started to menstruate, the girls had far more headaches and of much greater severity than the boys.

Monthly headaches seem to fall into three types—vacuum, tension, or migraine—according to Dr. Dalton.

The one termed a vacuum headache by Dr. Dalton is commonly called a sinus headache. But Dr. Dalton does not use this term because a true sinus headache is caused by an infection in one of the sinus cavities. A vacuum headache, however, produces the same sensations. It makes you feel that your nose is blocked. You find it hard to breathe through one or both nostrils. The pain that you may experience as pressure or tenderness is located in the sinus cavities—above the eyes, in the cheek bones, or on either side of the nose. A vacuum headache usually pains more when you bend over or when you turn your head suddenly.

A tension headache feels more like there is a tight steel band pressing in on your head, or a heavy weight sitting on top of your skull. The muscles in the neck are very tight and contracted. Many women complain of a stiff neck and have difficulty turning the head from side to side. Dr. Dalton has observed that most tension headaches appear in the days preceding menstruation and gradually fade away with the start of the menses.

"The pain of a migraine is like dozens of razor blades slashing the side of my head," says one sufferer. To another, "It is like a meteor slamming into my skull." And to someone else, "A migraine makes me feel that my brain is about to explode." Although most migraine attacks come just before menstruation, they sometimes occur during the menstrual period. Usually, migraines last between twenty-four and forty-eight hours. But some sufferers have reported migraines that persisted as long as ten days and actually required hospitalization.

A migraine can make you supersensitive to your surroundings. Bright lights, loud noises, strong smells, even a light touch, can be extremely painful. Foods may lose their taste and have to be highly seasoned to be enjoyed. Migraines are often accompanied by nausea and vomiting, chills and sweating, and exhaustion.

In the so-called classical migraine, the onset is marked by an aura, a warning signal that lasts for twenty minutes or more, when the victim sees flashing lights and/or bright stars, and feels dizzy. Common migraine sneaks up on the sufferer. It starts gradually, and slowly gains in intensity and severity.

BREAST TENDERNESS AND SWELLING

Sore, enlarged breasts are a common physical symptom of PMS. In fact, Dr. Michael G. Brush writes that if you have mild PMS, tender, swollen breasts may be your only complaint. At such times, a hug or any pressure on the breasts may be painful. Your bras feel too snug and much less comfortable than usual. Then, as soon as your period starts, everything returns to normal.

Sometimes women are afraid that their enlarged breasts are an indication of cancer or some other disease. There is no connection at all between the breast swelling of PMS and cancer.

WEIGHT GAIN
AND BLOATING

You may find, in the days before menstruation, that you show a weight gain and feel heavier than usual. The weight gain may be between three and seven pounds, although increases as great as fourteen pounds have been reported.

The weight increase and bloating are the results of the body's retention of water. Usually, excess water is eliminated from the body through urine and perspiration. Before menstruation, however, the water you have taken in through food and drink collects in a number of places around the body. When your period starts, the water-retention problem disappears. One woman reportedly gained twelve to fourteen pounds before each period. On the first day of menstruation, she lost it all, producing nine pints of urine.

Where the water accumulates before you menstruate depends on your particular physical makeup. Water may collect in your extremities, such as your ankles and feet or your arms and fingers. The extra water in the tissues of your lower extremities, for example, may make it hard for you to stand on your feet for long stretches of time. You may tire quickly if you walk for any distance. Shoes may feel unusually tight. If fingers swell, it may become hard to remove rings that otherwise slip on and off easily.

If the water collects in your abdomen, it can make your stomach swell and your waistline expand. Clothes that usually fit just fine now become very tight. Zippers on jeans are difficult to pull up; pants or skirts reveal stomach bulges in an unflattering way.

The natural reaction to feeling puffed up, or bloated, is to go on a diet. But it is best not to start a diet at this time. When your period starts, your tissues will release the water that has accumulated. The bulges and bloatedness will begin to go away.

Have you successfully followed a diet and then found that your weight suddenly and inexplicably increased? The weight gain could be a symptom of PMS. Do not think that your diet is not working and go on an eating binge. Remember that it may be a temporary condition that will end with the onset of menstruation.

CONSTIPATION

Constipation, that is, difficulty in moving your bowels, may occur before the menses begin. The fact is that constipation can also be a side effect of water retention.

The gynecologist Dr. Lucienne Lanson explains that there is a shift of fluid away from the bowel passageway to the walls of the intestine. This tends to make the stools somewhat drier than usual. With the start of your period, though, the fluid level adjusts itself. The constipation ends. For a day or two things may even swing the other way. You may have loose bowel movements before your system returns to normal.

SKIN DISORDERS

'My skin becomes pink and blotchy for about one week of every month," says one nineteen-year-old woman. "As soon as I get my period it clears up, and I'm fine for the next three weeks or so."

Skin problems such as pimples, boils, sties, cold sores, and acne are all common signs of PMS. Doctors have different opinions on the exact causes of skin changes before the period. But almost all agree that the eruptions have to do with the changes that are taking place in the body at that time.

Take acne, for example. Acne is caused by the accumulation of sebum, grease, in the pores. The production of sebum does not begin until puberty. Often it takes a few years for the body to become able to regulate the amount. Once this happens the acne disappears.

Estrogen plays an important part in slowing down the production of sebum. At times of falling levels of estrogen, the problem reappears. This may be at ovulation or before menstruation. The opposite effect occurs when estrogen levels are high. Few pregnant women or those on birth control pills suffer from acne.

ACHES AND PAINS

During the last week or so before menstruation begins, you wake up in the morning with a dull, heavy soreness in your lower abdomen. Or your back, knees, ankles, shoulders, hands, or hips suddenly begin to ache. The aches and pains keep getting worse. They never get quite bad enough to make you stay in bed. But they are an irritation. Then suddenly, on the first day of your period, they begin to taper off, and so do the other symptoms of PMS.

What is happening may be congestive dysmenorrhea—different from spasmodic dysmenorrhea, the pain that accompanies menstruation. The way to tell them apart is to notice when they occur. Congestive dysmenorrhea comes only before your menses, nearly each and every month. Spasmodic dysmenorrhea arrives with the onset of the menses, not before.

There are other differences between the two kinds

of menstrual pain, too. Generally, congestive dysmenorrhea is more severe when you are under stress. Also,
the aches and pains are more spread out and not always
in your lower abdomen and genital area, as with spasmodic dysmenorrhea. The differences become especially important when deciding on treatment. Opposite
kinds of therapies are needed for the two conditions.
The wrong treatment can worsen the symptoms.

ASTHMA

Dr. Katharina Dalton has found a close connection
between PMS and asthma, a condition marked by difficulty in breathing along with wheezing and coughing.
She reports that about one-third of all women between
puberty and menopause tend to have premenstrual
asthma attacks. The problem seems especially prevalent
in the very young and then again in the group over forty
years of age.

Usually, asthma is considered an allergic reaction.
But Dr. Dalton believes that premenstrual asthma may
have another origin altogether. The attack is usually
sudden and acute, often occurring in the middle of the
night. It may last a few hours or several days. Then,
with the beginning of menstruation, it suddenly stops.

EPILEPSY

Recent research by Dr. Richard H. Mattson, professor of
neurology at Yale University and a leader in the field,
pointed to a link between epilepsy and PMS. Epilepsy is
a condition in which a person's muscles contract suddenly, and there is a brief loss of consciousness. Dr.
Mattson found that certain women had attacks of epilepsy only in the week before menstruation. Often the
attacks followed the appearance of such other physical
symptoms as headaches.

You, or someone you know, may notice that epilepsy occurs only before the menstrual period. Or you may find that epileptic episodes are worse when they occur during that time. By correctly treating your PMS, you may stop the attacks or reduce their severity. In some cases, epileptic women who were being treated with anti-convulsive drugs no longer required medication.

EYE PROBLEMS

Conjunctivitis and glaucoma are two eye disorders that appear to have some connection with PMS. Conjunctivitis, also called pink eye, is usually caused by an infection. But Dr. Dalton has also observed its monthly appearance in certain women during the premenstrual period.

Glaucoma is a condition in which the fluid pressure inside the eyeball increases. It can get so high that it can actually damage the optic nerve and cause blindness. At London's Institute of Ophthalmology, doctors found that 89 percent of women with glaucoma also suffered with PMS, and 60 percent experienced raised pressure during the premenstrual time of the month.

NOSE AND THROAT AILMENTS

One young woman who had monthly colds for years finally went to an alert doctor who recognized the colds as one of the premenstrual symptoms. Actually, many people who think they have some kind of flu, hoarseness, or hay fever, turn out to be experiencing PMS.

One entertainer always avoided auditions for singing dates the week before her menstrual period. She had learned that every month hoarseness made her voice deeper. She couldn't sing as high as usual. Eventually, she received treatment for her PMS, and the problem cleared up.

The loss of smell is a common symptom that many women have, but few may notice. A certain manufacturer of antiperspirants and deodorants had long been aware that some users tended to change brands every three or four weeks. When asked why, the women explained that they found the product was no longer effective. Research showed that the dissatisfaction was due to a combination of factors. Just before and during menses, the women showed a rise in perspiration and vaginal discharge. At the same time, their ability to smell the deodorant's perfume was diminished. Convinced that the product no longer worked, they switched brands.

CLUMSINESS AND POOR COORDINATION

During your premenstrual time, you may find that you drop things more often than usual, walk into furniture, knock over things. Probably, if you are like most people, you blame yourself for being clumsy and uncoordinated.

The reality is that many women with PMS tend to be more accident prone in the premenstrual days than at any other time. In fact, recent studies of a number of female athletes show a drop in their scores and abilities due to errors in performance before their period and in the first day or two of menstruation.

BRUISING, FAINTING, AND DIZZINESS

One of the most unusual symptoms of PMS is the appearance of "spontaneous" bruises. These are black-

and-blue marks that show up on your skin without your being able to remember any blow or injuries to those spots.

Even more annoying, and quite common in the days before menstruation, are fainting spells. Dr. Dalton notes that the incidence is highest among teenage girls who often skip breakfast and may have to stand in one place for a long time during the day. Dizziness is among the most frequent of the PMS symptoms. It is often worse when bending over or turning the head sharply, or while experiencing a headache. Women who have had children and are approaching menopause may find these symptoms growing more severe.

Perhaps as you read about the physical symptoms of PMS, you find that you do not have PMS or experience it only to a mild degree. Nevertheless, it is good to stay alert to the symptoms. Mild symptoms can be present for a number of years, and then there can be a sudden change. The symptoms may disappear all at once— or they may grow worse. Like all medical disorders, diagnosis is the first step to freeing yourself, and helping to free others, of the condition and the symptoms.

4

THE PSYCHOLOGICAL SYMPTOMS OF PMS

In the week or so before your period:
> Do you feel tense and depressed?
> Do you suffer anxiety or panic attacks?
> Do you feel unloved, irritable, and defensive?
> Do you lash out at others for little or no reason?
> Do you crave sweets, carbohydrates, salty foods, or alcohol?
> Do you cry easily, sometimes without reason?

When your period begins:
> Do you suddenly feel like an enormous cloud has lifted?
> Do you feel like your own self again?
> Are you better able to handle day-to-day problems and responsibilities?
> Do you have trouble recalling the way you felt and behaved?

If you said yes to some or all of the above questions, you may be among those suffering the psychological symptoms of PMS. Very possibly you never considered these symptoms part of any disorder; you just thought that it was part of your personality. Or the behavior patterns made you feel guilty, ashamed, and afraid at times that you were neurotic or even going mad.

A clear link between PMS and behavior has yet to be established. But an increase in such emotional discomfort before menstruation, and the absence of such symptoms after menstruation, is known in many women. The change also shows up as an increase in female suicides, admissions to psychiatric hospitals, and calls to psychiatric hot lines in the days before the start of menstruation.

TENSION

All of us get tense at one time or another. A crucial moment in a ball game, the sight of a crime or accident, an important test, or a job interview—any one of these situations can make you trembly, unable to draw a deep breath, and generally uptight. But in some women an attack of tension comes on very suddenly and without apparent cause during the premenstrual period.

Frequently it feels like the tension we experience at other times, except that there is nothing happening to set it off. Sometimes it is more acute and lasts longer. One woman says, "I can't stop talking for days on end. Various thoughts, accusations, verbal abuses keep pouring out of my mouth. I know I'm being hateful and unfair, but I can't seem to calm down."

Tension is believed to underlie many of the symptoms of PMS. For example, clumsiness, which often increases in the premenstrual period, may originate in a lack of concentration due to tension. Asthma and epileptic attacks, too, can sometimes be triggered by increased tension. And some believe that tiredness and fatigue may be nothing more than the body's response to a high level of tension.

Like some other symptoms of PMS, stress in the days before menstruation can make matters a lot worse. The individual becomes more anxious and fearful. About one half of all the mothers who bring children to hospital emergency rooms or doctors' offices do it during their premenstrual period. This may well be because they are least able to cope with the children's illnesses at this time.

IRRITABILITY

There is a story about a husband who, sensing his wife's difficulty with PMS, brought her a bouquet of flowers. Instead of appreciating his gesture, in a sudden fit of irritability she flung the flowers to the floor, called them a stupid waste of money, and slapped his face. Then, the next day, when he did not bring her any present, she berated him for being so thoughtless and uncaring! Too often husbands and wives do not associate edginess and agitation with the premenstrual phase of the menstrual cycle. Some experts believe that not only husband abuse, but also wife beatings, may be triggered by behavior caused by premenstrual irritability.

Perhaps children suffer most keenly. There exist many tragic accounts of mothers who are gentle and loving most of the time, but who lose control of themselves in the days before menstruation. They may beat and otherwise injure their children. One thirty-year-old mother of two young children said, "Just before my last period, I became very angry at my three-year-old daughter. I threw her down very hard on the floor. Afterwards, I couldn't stop crying and feeling guilty. I would never have thought myself capable of doing such a terrible thing."

Loss of temper and violent outbursts may start at puberty or after the birth of children. They are a recurring theme in many accounts of women who commit violent crimes. Some recent surveys show that among women prisoners, 50 percent in London, 62 percent in New York City, and 84 percent in Paris had committed their crimes within four days of their period. Of course it is not too surprising that sudden, explosive demonstrations of irritability or aggression may result in arrests and jailings. But it is also possible that lack of alertness, slower reactions, and poor concentration make the criminals more apt to be caught.

Many adolescents with PMS handle their mental distress by acting out, threatening suicide, and abusing alcohol and/or drugs. Sometimes these monthly spells of irritability alternate with happy and joyful times. But when one sixteen-year-old became extremely difficult, she was expelled from school. Not long after, she became involved with heroin and other dangerous drugs. She was arrested repeatedly for shoplifting, burglary, and a number of other offenses. It was only after several years in and out of jail that she became aware that every one of her arrests came within days before her period. With the help of a women's self-help group, she was able to control her PMS, and has now returned to school to finish her education.

DEPRESSION

From "feeling blue" to wanting to commit suicide, depression is the most common complaint of all women. According to some experts, as many as 85 percent of all females experience depression. The signs of depression—moodiness; little pleasure or interest in activity, people, or events; lack of energy; crying jags; lack of concentration; forgetfulness; insomnia—usually occur between ovulation and menstruation. Often the symptoms are not too severe. You may just feel that you are not quite yourself for a few days. Then, once menstruation begins, you are back to normal.

Dr. Ronald V. Norris estimates that about 30 percent of women with severe PMS suffer, in addition, from clinical depression. Clinical depression is a chronic condition that does not stop with the onset of menstruation. It does not occur just now and again. It persists most of the time and pervades all facets of life.

Depression is not always diagnosed properly. Some doctors may recognize it as part of PMS and treat it accordingly. With treatment, the depression often disappears. But in women suffering from PMS as well as clinical depression, a treatment that includes psychotherapy is needed. Treatment for PMS alone will not eliminate the depression.

In serious cases, depression can lead to suicide. In fact, the premenstrual phase has been found to be the time of most suicide attempts. A study of attempted suicides by hospitalized women in Los Angeles, London, and Delhi (India) shows that as many as 50 percent occurred in the four days before or after menstruation.

TIREDNESS

Tiredness seems to be closely tied to depression. Overall feelings of fatigue and lethargy usually accompany depression. You know that you are tired when you don't have the energy to carry out your daily routine. Given your choice, you would spend the whole day in bed, doing nothing.

Dr. Dalton believes that tiredness leads to an apparent reduction in mental ability during the premenstrual period. In one study of the grades of 1,561 girls in an English boarding school, she found that most were "normal" during the second and third weeks of their menstrual cycles. During the premenstrual week, though, their grades dropped about 10 percent, and during the following week, they jumped up 20 percent.

Curiously enough, if tiredness is part of your PMS, you may find that it is preceded by an amazing burst of energy. Perhaps on that one day you jog five miles, clean out your closets, and catch up on your correspondence. A day or two later, you enter the premenstrual phase and feel washed out and listless. If you are not aware of the PMS, you may blame the fatigue on over-exertion.

ALCOHOLISM

A recent survey of women alcoholics in America reveals that PMS may pose a triple threat for this group. Fully two-thirds of the women said that they could not control their heavy drinking just before menstruation, although they could the rest of the time.

All said that their drinking problem had started or grown more serious the week or so before menstruation. The fact is that alcohol tolerance drops during the premenstrual phase. A woman who usually can have two or three drinks without feeling the effects, becomes drunk on half the amount during this time period.

Finally, premenstrual drinking sprees tend to become habit forming, even addictive. In the words of one patient, "I started to drink during my premenstrual time because I felt so bad. Sipping Scotch made my aches and pains dissolve. Before I knew it, though, I needed another drink, and then another. Soon it took a whole pint of liquor to make me feel good."

Alcohol strikes some women with PMS as the perfect solution. The initial effect is to calm tension and soothe anxiety. It relieves the distress, gives pleasure, and makes the individual feel important. Also, it generally alters reality so that problems become less demanding. Conflicts seem easier to control.

But alcohol is a mind-altering substance, just like any drug. It has a general depressant effect on the central nervous system. For someone with PMS, who may already be depressed, the alcohol usually intensifies the despair and worsens the sense of hopelessness. Also, many people combine alcohol with other kinds of drugs, legal and illegal. According to Dr. Norris, women over forty who drink a lot tend to combine its use with drugs.

FOOD CRAVINGS

You may have heard that pregnant women crave certain foods. But did you know that a craving for sweets, such as chocolate, ice cream, and sodas, as well as a very strong desire for salty foods, is a frequent sign of PMS?

A recent study by Drs. Stuart Smith and Cynthia Sander of Canada, among many other studies, supports this point. In a sample group of 300 nurses, they found "a rather striking association" between PMS, depression, and a craving for sweets in the premenstrual period.

In some cases, doctors find that the food craving goes beyond the extra sweets some feel they must have at this time. It may lead to excessive eating of all foods or binge eating, a sudden and compulsive need to eat a lot in a very short time.

Some people feel almost powerless to resist this urge. As one woman put it, "I eat enough for a whole week in just one meal." Someone else told Dr. Dalton that one night, after going to bed, some force led her to the kitchen. In quick order she consumed two loaves of bread with peanut butter, a box of ginger cookies, and an apple tart!

At Dr. Norris's PMS clinic in Massachusetts, most patients are overweight. They have trouble staying on diets. Often they show wide fluctuations in weight. As many as 80 percent indulge in binge eating during the premenstrual phase. The doctor's studies show that the weight gain in these women may be as little as three to five pounds in small binges; in extreme cases, up to fifteen pounds. Unlike the gain due to water retention, this added weight does not disappear at the start of menstruation. Often the only real solution is a sound nutritional program with daily exercises.

How tense, irritable, depressed, tired, or dependent on alcohol and foods you feel in your premenstrual period depends very much on your personality and life style. The way you feel at other times of the month and the severity of your physical problems affect the kinds of psychological changes you may undergo.

Once again, the importance of recognizing your symptoms needs to be stressed. If most of your symptoms are psychological, discuss them with your family. Let them understand what you are going through each month. Then, when you burst out crying for no reason or have a sudden temper tantrum, they will be less likely to get upset or irritated. Aware of your symptoms, they can support you in your efforts to cope better.

5

CAUSES
OF PMS

Linda and Jane are the same age, height, and weight. Both are healthy and normal in all respects. But Linda has PMS, and Jane does not. Why?

The fact is that no one really knows. What causes PMS in some women but not in others is still under study. But thanks to recent research, scientists now have many theories and new insights as to why certain women experience the symptoms of PMS while others do not.

HORMONAL PROBLEMS

The most popular theory comes from Dr. Dalton. She finds much evidence to suggest that PMS is caused by a deficiency of progesterone in relation to the amount of estrogen in the blood between ovulation and menstruation. As you will recall, the production of the two female sex hormones, estrogen and progesterone, plays a vital role in the menstrual cycle. Normally, estrogen is produced in great quantities during the first part of the cycle; in the second phase both estrogen and progesterone are produced.

Among the many factors that Dr. Dalton has found to support her theory of progesterone deficiency are the following:

> 1. PMS only appears before menstruation, when progesterone should be in the woman's system; the symptoms vanish after menstruation, when progesterone is usually at a very low level.
> 2. PMS usually starts at puberty, after childbirth, or after stopping the regular use of birth-control pills—times of lowered progesterone in the blood.
> 3. PMS rarely appears during pregnancy, when progesterone production is very high.
> 4. PMS sufferers do not have the same steady rise in body temperature after ovulation as do other women, and it is believed that they do not because of an insufficient amount of progesterone.
> 5. Women with PMS tend to have lower levels of progesterone after ovulation than those without the symptoms.

Given these factors, Dr. Dalton would now like to find the reasons for the lack of progesterone in relation to the estrogen. What causes this hormonal imbalance? Is the ovary responsible for the poor production of the hormone? Is it lack of LH from the pituitary? A combination of factors?

Any disturbance in hormonal balance can produce the symptoms we associate with PMS. Levels of progesterone and estrogen affect your mood, whether you feel irritable or depressed, tense or anxious. They also can affect water retention in the body and bloatedness.

Until very recently doctors were not able to measure the presence of particular hormones in the blood with any great accuracy. It was especially difficult to track down progesterone, which is added to the blood stream in spurts. But a new technique, called radioimmunoassay, although still difficult and expensive to use, is now available for this purpose.

One of the most striking findings on hormonal imbalance comes from an experiment conducted in 1977 on 100 women with PMS at St. Thomas's Hospital in London. Using radioimmunoassay, Professor R. W. Taylor and Dr. Michael G. Brush found nearly half had levels of progesterone below the normal levels during the second part of the menstrual cycle.

About the same number, however, had more estrogen than expected. Excess estrogen accompanied by normal levels of progesterone also seemed to produce the symptoms. A higher-than-normal level of estrogen, especially, can make the breasts tender, swollen, and sore. Estrogen excess with too little progesterone had a similar effect. The conclusion seemed to be that it is the balance between the two hormones that is crucial. Any upset in this balance—too much estrogen or too little progesterone—can cause PMS.

A few women in the same study had "high-normal" or above-normal levels of prolactin (another hormone produced by the pituitary gland) in their blood. Too high a level of this hormone can interfere with the ovaries' production of estrogen and progesterone. Dr. Dalton suggests that excessive prolactin may be responsible for progesterone deficiency. Prolactin, Dr. Dalton believes, affects the breasts. This may explain why women with high levels of prolactin frequently have tender, enlarged breasts before the onset of their period.

While hormonal imbalances occur in women with PMS, no one knows why. Could it be due to heredity, some factor passed from mother to daughter? Is it due to change in life style from continual childbearing in the past to few pregnancies in most women today? Why is it not present in every woman? Why do some sufferers have normal hormonal balance? Could something else be involved?

Researchers are now devising special tests to explore further progesterone deficiency and hormonal imbalance as the main causes of PMS. Thus far more doctors administer progesterone to patients with severe PMS than any other treatment.

WATER RETENTION

During the premenstrual period, the normal excretion of water from the body undergoes some changes. Scientists believe that the estrogen produced by the ovaries retains extra amounts of the sodium found in salt. The sodium binds the water in the body, and as a result less water is eliminated through the kidneys.

What happens to the excess water if it is not eliminated? The water filters into the body's various cells and tissues. It may make you feel heavy and bloated. If water collects in the chambers of the eyes, for example, a buildup of pressure can hurt the eye (glaucoma). Some experts contend that water retention in the tissue cells of the brain may be at least partly responsible for triggering attacks of epilepsy.

When water builds up in the cells at the entrance to the sinuses, according to Dr. Dalton, you may suffer a vacuum headache. If the cells in the lungs are affected, you may find it difficult to breathe. Swelling in the nasal passages can produce the symptoms of a cold or hay fever. You may even lose your sense of smell. Swollen tissues in the inner ear can bring on attacks of dizziness.

Many, but not all, investigators blame fluid retention for the symptoms of PMS. Some recent studies show that not all women with PMS experience this interference with normal excretion of urine. At least one scientist suggests that it is just a symptom, not a basic cause of PMS.

LOW BLOOD SUGAR

You may think that a craving for sweets in the week or so before your period is purely psychological. You feel depressed and uncomfortable, so you reward yourself with something good to eat that will make you feel better. A number of studies, though, suggest that the food cravings may be physical in origin. You have a real need for candy, chocolate, ice cream, or some other source of sugar.

Normally, your blood-sugar level rises quickly each time that you eat. The level gradually drops until you eat again. As long as you eat before five hours have elapsed, or overnight before thirteen hours have gone by, your blood sugar stays within the normal range. But what happens if no food is taken for a very long time? Your blood sugar continues to fall until it reaches a critical level, called the base line. When that point is reached, your body sends out a spurt of the hormone adrenalin. The adrenalin releases some of the sugar that is stored in your body, and the blood sugar rises to a safe level.

Between ovulation and menstruation, changes may occur in the hormone levels that seem to affect sugar tolerance. The base line rises. Your body requires a higher level of blood sugar than at other times. Therefore, you need to take in more sugar to stay in the normal range. That is why you crave something sweet. If you don't get it, the adrenalin appears. You may experience headaches, irritability, feelings of panic, weakness, fainting or chills—common reactions to the sudden appearance of adrenalin, the "fight or flee" hormone.

Being aware that food craving is one of your symptoms of PMS may not stop you from eating a little extra in the days before your period. But with treatment, you should be able to control your craving. And you can learn which foods are best to avoid and which are best to eat.

VITAMIN DEFICIENCY

Since the 1940s, various experts have suspected that estrogen excess in PMS was the result of a vitamin-B-complex deficiency. When treated with these vitamins, PMS sufferers seemed to improve. Further research shows that a B-vitamin deficiency may affect liver function in women with PMS. The inability of the liver to break down estrogen may lead to the excess of estrogen in the blood.

The menstrual cycle, you will recall, is controlled by the function of the hypothalamus and the pituitary. In order for these brain structures to function properly, certain substances must be circulating in the blood. One of these substances, most doctors agree, is vitamin B_6, or pyridoxine. Pyridoxine has been found to lessen the symptoms of severe PMS, though it's not clear why.

Pyridoxine is believed necessary for the normal functioning of the hypothalamus and the central nervous system. Like other vitamins in the B-complex group, pyridoxine is vital to sound physical and emotional health. It helps to metabolize fats and carbohydrates and to break down proteins. Some claim that it maintains the production of such important hormones as estrogen and progesterone and such pituitary hormones as FSH and LH.

A lack of pyridoxine may affect the nervous system—the condition of nerves, stress, moods, and the general state of the emotions. A reduced supply of the vitamin may be responsible for depression. Below-average levels of pyridoxine can lead to adverse effects on the ovaries and breasts, and possibly induce fluid retention.

No large-scale, carefully planned research projects have yet determined whether or not the lack of B_6, or any other vitamin, is responsible for PMS. Scientists believe that more research is needed. Drs. Robert L. Reid and S.S.C. Yen of the University of California, San Diego, suggest a remote possibility that a cyclic vitamin deficiency exists in women who have PMS.

OTHER POSSIBLE CAUSES OF PMS

One of the oldest theories is that PMS is psychological in origin. Such eminent figures in the mental health field as Sigmund Freud and Karl Menninger have held this view. These authorities studied mother-daughter and father-daughter relationships at various stages of development, seeking possible sources of negative attitudes. Based on their findings, if you are unprepared for menstruation, jealous of your father or brother, confused about your sexual identity, conflicted over being female, the result may be PMS.

Although no one knows why, PMS does appear to run in families. "I've got it; my sister and mother have it, too," says one seventeen-year-old. The incidence among close relatives seems too high to be just coincidence. In cases of twins, for example, both Dr. Dalton in England and Dr. Norris in America have observed that twins *always* have the identical symptoms of PMS, at just about the same level of intensity. And the twin sisters develop the symptoms at about the same time in life, too.

41

Supporters of the theory that PMS is transmitted at birth cite the fact that many women show PMS at puberty. Certain risk factors, they believe, trigger the signal in the genes to produce the symptoms. Opponents of the theory argue that PMS appears among close relatives because all of us tend to mimic the behaviors of those with whom we live. Also, they say, there are many families in which just one woman in each generation shows the traits of PMS. What is needed is research to track the genetic traits of PMS through many generations of mothers, daughters, and sisters.

The theory of hormone allergy as a cause of PMS originated back in 1921. Dr. J. Gerber collected samples of blood from PMS subjects during their premenstrual phase. Later, when they were no longer in this phase, he injected them with the serum. The serum brought on some of the same PMS symptoms.

In the mid-1940s, Drs. B. Zondek and Y. M. Bromberg first stated the idea that some symptoms of PMS might be the body's allergic reaction to the hormones produced during the premenstrual period. Other investigators tried to make patients less sensitive to a certain hormone by giving them daily injections of increasing amounts. Although the experiment was flawed, it did relieve the symptoms of PMS in some 80 percent of the subjects.

Certain foods seem to contribute greatly to the migraine headaches associated with PMS. The most common foods that you may be sensitive to are cheese, chocolate, alcohol, and citrus fruits. Lower down on the list are ripe bananas, pork, onion, and fish.

With migraine, in the menstrual phase, you may find that the attack does not come right after the food has been eaten. Usually, the reaction occurs between twelve and thirty-six hours later. Dr. Dalton suggests that something happens when the digested food reaches the liver. If a special chemical is not present, a malfunction occurs. The result is that substances are released that are able to open wide the blood vessels of the brain, which may trigger the headache. The various substances are formed from the breakdown of the foods we mentioned earlier. But finding which foods cause your PMS reaction is up to you. Often this kind of sensitivity runs in families. Perhaps some relatives can point out the foods that produce their PMS. That can help you pinpoint the ones that cause you trouble.

One of the very latest theories of PMS is that it springs from a disturbance in the body's neurotransmitters. Neurotransmitters are chemicals that transmit signals from one nerve cell to another in the brain. Proposed by Drs. Reid and Yen in 1981, this theory suggests that there may be problems present in the neurotransmitters involved with the control of the menstrual cycle. These difficulties become magnified many times over as the hypothalamus, pituitary, ovaries, and uterus become involved.

If you think you have PMS, you should pay attention first to the most widely accepted causes of the disorder—hormonal imbalance, fluid retention, low blood sugar, and vitamin deficiency. Then, take a careful look at the other possibilities and consider them carefully.

Much research remains to be done. Well-designed experiments have to be run on large numbers of subjects. This will put the various theories to the test. Answers to important questions must be found: Is PMS a single condition, or a combination of several disorders that just happen tó appear together? Is there a single cause for PMS or more than one?

6

SELF-HELP
FOR PMS

Have you heard the good-news bad-news story as it
applies to the various treatments for PMS? First, the bad
news. There's no single treatment and method that
works for everyone. Now the good news. There *are*
ways to relieve most of the symptoms; about 80 percent
of women with PMS are successfully treated.

If you know or suspect that you have PMS, what
does this mean for you? It means that you have an excellent chance of bringing most, if not all, of the bother-
some symptoms under control. It also suggests that in
all but the most serious cases, you can deal with PMS by
yourself. Many women with mild to moderate PMS
have improved their condition without any medical
help.

KEEPING A CHART

To be sure that your symptoms occur in a regular
monthly pattern—a week or ten days before your peri-

od, and no symptoms after that—you need to keep a chart for several months. The chart will do several things for you. It will help you decide if you have PMS. It will help you understand your own menstrual cycle. It will zero in on your particular symptoms. And if all else fails and you decide to go for medical help, it will tell a doctor a lot about your condition.

You may prepare a three-month chart on a piece of lined notebook paper. Number the lines 1 through 31 (draw extra lines, if necessary). They represent the days of the month. Divide the rest of the page into three columns. Head the first column with the name of the current month; the others with the names of the following two months.

Once you begin, you will enter four bits of information in the slot next to the proper day of the month. First, you will enter your body temperature, taken as soon as you wake up in the morning (for example, 97.9°). Called the basal temperature readings, and taken with a special thermometer called an Ovalindex or basal body temperature thermometer, the figures will help you to understand the timing of your symptoms. When you ovulate, your temperature rises about one degree and stays there until your next menstrual period. Later, by looking at the temperature and the symptoms, you can decide if your symptoms are truly premenstrual.

The second item you need to enter in the same slot is your nude weight on rising. Dr. Norris suggests emptying your bladder before stepping on the scale. If the weight gain disappears after your period, you will know that you are probably retaining water in the premenstrual phase. On the other hand, if you put on weight due to binge eating, you will probably not lose it unless you diet.

Thirdly, you will want to enter any symptoms you experience day by day. This suggested code may help record the physical symptoms:

A—Asthma
Ba—Back Pain
Bl—Bloating
Br—Breast Tenderness
Bru—Bruising
C—Clumsiness
D—Dizziness
E—Eye Problems
Fa—Fainting
Fd—Food Binges
H—Headaches
N—Nausea
Sk—Skin Disorders
Sz—Seizures
Wt—Weight Gain

The psychological signs may be indicated in the following way:
Al—Alcoholism
Ag—Aggressiveness
An—Anxiety
Cr—Crying Jags
De—Depression
I—Irritability
L—Lethargy
M—Moodiness
Su—Suicidal Thoughts
Te—Tension
Ti—Tiredness

You can make each entry even more accurate and helpful by indicating the severity of the symptoms. In addition to the letter symbol for each symptom, rank them 1 (mild), 2 (moderate), or 3 (severe). You may want to ask a family member or close friend whom you see daily to help you with the symptom entries. You may not always be the best judge of your physical reactions or mental behavior.

The fourth kind of information you enter has to do with your actual menstrual period, from onset to last day of bleeding, indicated by the circled letter M. If you have PMS, you should be able to detect a pattern of symptoms occurring in the days before your period, followed by completely symptom-free days right after your period ends.

When you are finished, your daily chart for one month might resemble the one on page 49.

THE DAILY REPORT

On the days you suffer the most, you can also keep a kind of diary. This personal account will give some detailed information. Here is an example:

Date: June 17

Symptoms and degree of severity:

Awoke feeling confused and angry. Had desperate need to be alone. Did not want to talk to anyone! Body feels bloated. If only everyone would leave me alone, I might just get by.

Foods eaten and times:
Skipped breakfast
Lunch—Two slices of pizza and soda; candy bar
Dinner—Spaghetti and meatballs, cole slaw, chocolate cake

Special happenings:
Failed English final. Had fight with boy friend. Told him I never want to see him again. Went for walk, and began to feel better.

A number of daily reports of the premenstrual phase can point up an association between the time of the

SEPTEMBER	OCTOBER	NOVEMBER
1. 97.9° 105		
2. 97.9 105		
3. 98.0 105		
4. 97.9 105		
5. 98.1 105		
6. 97.9 105		
7. 98.1 105		
8. 97.8 105		
9. 97.9 105		
10. 97.8 105		
11. 97.8 105		
12. 98.2 105		
13. 98.5 105		
14. 98.9 106 De-1, I-1		
15. 98.8 107 De-2		
16. 98.6 108 De-2		
17. 98.4 109 De-2, H-3		
18. 98.5 110 De-1, H-3, Bl-3		
19. 98.5 110 De-1, Bl-2, Fd-2		
20. 98.5 110 De-2, Bl-2, Fd-2		
21. 98.5 110 De-1, Bl-1, Fd-2		
22. 98.4 109 De-1, Bl-2		
23. 98.4 109 De-1, Bl-2		
24. 98.0 108 Ⓜ		
25. 97.9 107 Ⓜ		
26. 97.6 106 Ⓜ		
27. 97.2 105 Ⓜ		
28. 97.2 105 Ⓜ		
29. 97.6 105		
30. 97.9 105		
31.		

cycle, symptoms, effect of stress and anxiety, and influence of pleasurable activities on PMS.

EATING WELL

All medical researchers on PMS agree on one thing—skipping meals, eating like a bird, or consuming a lot of sweets can worsen the symptoms of PMS. In fact, if you are like many people, you may cut back on food when you are feeling tense and unhappy. The lack of food at a time when your body sorely needs nourishment can be particularly bad for you.

Whether or not you have PMS, you should eat a well-balanced diet. Diet is the key to your well-being. That means you should get a good daily combination of vitamins, carbohydrates, proteins, and fats. Grains, such as wheat and rice, as well as nuts, seeds, and pasta of all kinds are especially good for you when you have the symptoms of PMS. That is because these foods provide carbohydrates of the slow-burning variety needed for energy, not the refined sugars that are responsible for the sudden rise and fall in the level of blood sugar. It is also recommended that you eat six small meals a day rather than three large ones.

Vegetables and salads are excellent for meeting your daily nutritional needs and for keeping you filled up. This is particularly important at a time when you seem always to be hungry and concerned about weight gain. Naturally-sweet fruits should be eaten in moderate amounts because large quantities can bring on the same symptoms as refined sugars do.

As an added way to combat PMS tiredness, try to increase your intake of potassium during your premenstrual phase. Nuts, bananas, oranges, tomatoes, and soybeans are good sources of this important mineral. Potassium is also vital because it works together with sodium to maintain the balance of fluids in the body.

COMBATING SYMPTOMS OF PMS THROUGH DIET

Symptoms	Recommended	Some Sources	
Acne and Other Skin Disorders	Vitamin A	Apricots Carrots Eggs Milk	Peaches Pumpkins Sweet Potatoes
	Zinc	Eggs Fish	Red Meat
Tiredness	Potassium	Bananas Nuts Oranges	Tomatoes Soybeans
	Protein	Cheese Chicken Eggs	Fish Milk Yogurt

Water Retention	Diuretics	Cucumbers
		Parsley
		Watercress
		Watermelon
			Herbal Teas:
			  Chamomile
			  Dandelion
			  Thyme

Symptoms	To Be Avoided	Some Sources	
Fluid Retention	Salt	Beets Ham & Bacon Hot Dogs Mustard	Potato Chips Pretzels Sauerkraut Sausage
Irritability and Headaches	Caffeine	Chocolate Milk Cocoa	Coffee Soda Tea
Mood Swings	Refined Sugars	Cake Candy Chocolate	Ice Cream Soda

Water retention is a common symptom of potassium deficiency as are low blood sugar and fatigue.

High-protein foods are especially important in your diet if you feel tired and need more energy. Milk, eggs, cheese, and yogurt are excellent sources of both calcium and protein. Chicken and fish are rich in protein, but some people feel better when they eat meat in reasonable amounts during the premenstrual time. Doctors, you will recall, believe that pyridoxine (vitamin B_6) plays a role during the menstrual cycle. Therefore, it is wise to include foods particularly rich in B_6 as well as the other B vitamins, such as liver, milk, eggs, bran cereal, whole wheat bread, rice, and yeast.

To reduce the body's water content, it is wise to include certain foods whose diuretic properties help eliminate excess water from your tissues. Cucumber, watermelon, watercress, and parsley are mild natural diuretics. Herbal teas made with raspberry leaves, marjoram, thyme, dandelion leaves, or chamomile have the same effect. All reduce the swelling and bloatedness that result from water retention.

Vitamin therapy is also helpful in treating premenstrual flare-up of acne and other skin outbreaks. Some doctors recommend increasing your intake of vitamin A and zinc. Vitamin A is found in milk, butter, cheese, and eggs. Your body can also make vitamin A from carrots, sweet potatoes, pumpkins, peaches, and apricots. There is evidence that the body needs more zinc when it is under stress than at other times. Also, zinc is believed to be important to hormone metabolism. Seafood, meat, and eggs are good sources of zinc. You get little zinc from processed foods.

AVOIDING CERTAIN FOODS

Chief among the substances that can make you feel worse during the premenstrual period are those that contain refined sugars. Cake, candy, chocolate, ice cream, and soda are some prime examples. Sugar triggers the production of great amounts of insulin, a hormone that lowers the blood sugar level too fast or too much. Doctors suggest that you try to get over the idea of giving yourself a treat with sweets when you feel low. This may be difficult at first. But, in the long run, it will make you feel a whole lot better, both physically and emotionally.

Try to substitute so-called complex carbohydrates for foods rich in refined sugar. Eat whole-grain breads, cereals, and pasta products; beans; peas; oats; and wheat germ instead of highly processed foods which have sugar added to them. Most complex carbohydrates are digested and absorbed more slowly than sugar foods. They don't lead to the big swings in blood sugar that you get from sweet "junk foods." Being off sweets for a few months may relieve any extreme menstrual symptoms that you may have.

You may control fluid retention, in the days prior to menstruation, by eliminating salt from your diet. Salt contains sodium, which binds water in the body. Studies show women who experience weight gain and swelling of the hands, feet, or breasts in the premenstrual phase can reduce the symptoms by giving up salt and salty foods. "The first month, I gave up all sodium, and the effect was phenomenal!" said one young PMS sufferer. To name a few, foods high in salt include potato chips and pretzels, hot dogs and sausage, ham and bacon, mustard and ketchup, beets and sauerkraut.

If you are in the habit of drinking coffee, tea, soda, cocoa, or chocolate milk, you are getting a big dose of caffeine in your diet. Taking headache tablets, stay-awake pills, antacids, and some painkillers, adds even more of this substance. Although more research is needed, evidence suggests that caffeine may make certain symptoms of PMS worse.

Some believe that caffeine depletes the body's supply of B vitamins. Irritability and headaches seem to increase with the use of caffeine. Many PMS sufferers have found, therefore, that avoiding all foods with caffeine, even decaffeinated coffee, improves the way they feel, to varying degrees. Breast tenderness is thought to be related to a combination of too much caffeine and too little vitamin E. Insufficient vitamin E seems to be responsible for some menstrual disorders. Women with premenstrual problems are therefore advised, in addition to giving up caffeine, to increase their intake of lettuce, whole grains, meat, milk, and eggs—all good sources of vitamin E.

Headaches during the premenstrual days appear to be triggered by foods other than those with caffeine. Aged cheeses, such as cheddar and Parmesan; salami and bologna; red wine; ripe bananas; and avocados can be troublesome as well. Some people get bad headaches after eating figs, citrus fruit, nitrates, monosodium glutamate, tomatoes, or peanuts, or drinking alcohol or milk. If you are headache-prone, try giving up all these foods. Then reintroduce them one at a time to try to find out which ones are causing your headaches.

When you are premenstrual, and when you are not, you will probably feel better if you follow some basic principles of good nutrition:

1. Eat whole grains, nuts, and seeds instead of refined sugars and flours.
2. Avoid all beverages with caffeine, such as coffee, teas, soda (even decaffeinated coffees or teas).
3. Eat plenty of vegetables and fruits and relatively small quantities of meat, chicken, fish.
4. When hungry between meals, snack on milk, nuts, raisins. Eat several small meals a day, if possible, instead of two or three large meals.

EXERCISE
AND RELAXATION
TECHNIQUES

Most experimental evidence shows that women who are in good physical condition generally suffer fewer and milder PMS symptoms than those who are not. Tension and depression especially seem to be controlled by a regular exercise regime. One study of athletes and professional dancers shows that this group experienced far less tension and depression than others. Relieving tension through activity seems to make individuals less likely to have headaches, cramps, or feelings of tiredness or irritability.

Exercise helps provide a sense of well-being by improving blood circulation, increasing lung capacity, and controlling weight. But did you know that it also affects the functioning of the menstrual cycle? Recent research suggests that exercise may improve the production of neurotransmitters and hormones, such as progesterone. Vigorous exercise suppresses your appetite, sometimes for hours. And exercise causes the brain to release a natural tranquilizing chemical, beta-endorphin, resulting in the relief of tension.

Regular exercise means a minimum of fifteen to thirty minutes of vigorous activity at least three times a week all year long. If you are already in quite good physical condition and follow some kind of mild exercise program, you might want to advance to more strenuous activities, such as aerobic dancing, jogging, bicycling, or other sports. On the other hand, if you are overweight or very reluctant to do physical activity, you might want to start with a modest exercise program.

You should work yourself into condition *slowly*. Brisk walking, breathing deeply and slowly as you go, is usually a good way for beginners to start. Take short walks at first. Gradually increase the distances you cover and the speed. Set an early goal of a one-mile brisk walk five days a week.

Swimming exercises are good for relaxing all muscles, especially those of the uterus, and removing tension from the arms and legs. If you do not have access to a pool, you can do calisthenics several times a week at home. Specific exercises can remove muscle weakness that is related to back pain and such symptoms of tension as headaches.

Here is one good back exercise you can try: Lie flat on the floor. Contract your stomach. Press the small of your back against the floor. Relax. Repeat ten times.

To relax tension in your neck and shoulders: Stand, feet together, with arms at your sides. Drop your head down so your chin rests on your chest. Rotate your head slowly to the right side. To the back. To the left side. To the front. Repeat five times. Now rotate in the other direction. Repeat five times.

The particular type of exercise you choose to do depends on your age, weight, physical condition, and interests. The choice is yours. But once you embark on an exercise regimen, stick to it. Before long you may join the millions who are hooked on jogging, dancing, yoga, or whatever. One young woman says, "On days when I cannot exercise, I crash. I get intense feelings of irritability and unhappiness."

MANAGING STRESS

Stress in the premenstrual period, most everyone agrees, worsens the symptoms of PMS. As Dr. Norris points out, both the hypothalamus and the pituitary, which are concerned with the production of sex hormones, are also involved with our responses to stress. Major stress combined with the physical changes during the premenstrual period can exhaust the body. It affects such important processes as the body's retention of sodium, to take one example.

Finding your own way to reduce stress can help you lessen such symptoms as bloating and headaches. Some women find that going for walks, listening to music, taking hot baths, doing strenuous exercise, or watching television provides relief from stress. For others, meditation or yoga are relaxing, both physically and mentally. Hypnosis is successful for some women. And getting extra rest can be very helpful.

One popular way to reduce tension is through a system known as progressive relaxation. Wear comfortable clothes and no shoes. To get started, lie down on a rug or mat on the floor. Close your eyes. Imagine that you are on a warm, sandy beach. Consciously try to loosen your whole body. Imagine melting your body into the sand. When you feel relaxed, bend your hand up from the wrist. Notice the feeling that you get in your arm. That feeling is tension. Now let your hand drop down loosely. This feeling is relaxation. Repeat with your left hand, sensing the tension and relaxation.

Raise your right foot and feel the tension. Then lower it, and feel the relaxation. Repeat with the other foot.

Now practice tightening and loosening the various sets of muscles in your body. In progression, contract and relax the muscles in your legs, thighs, buttocks, abdomen, chest, shoulders, neck, face, eyes, tongue. For each set of muscles: tighten, count slowly to three, relax. Let the tension drain away. Rest a few seconds. Repeat five times.

It will only take about fifteen minutes every day to complete the relaxation exercises. After a while, you will be able to reach the goal of all who practice progressive relaxation. You will be able to relax the muscles of your body without tensing them first. You'll know you're at that stage when you lie down and within minutes feel completely relaxed from head to toe.

TALKING IT OUT

PMS is not only a personal problem. Your mood swings, temper tantrums, crying spells, accidents, lack of coordination, and other difficulties usually involve other members of your family. Talking about PMS with parents and friends can help them to know and understand you better. What's more, it can help them decide, during your difficult times, whether you need them to step in or to leave you alone.

Talking things over with other women who have symptoms of PMS can give you further ideas on how to handle your own situation. Since the 1970s, many women's support groups have formed to deal with a full range of feminist issues. These concerns include health problems such as PMS.

Find out if there is such a group where you live. (You will find a list of organizations in the back of this book.) If there is no such place to meet in your town or city, you might think about forming your own group. A list of national organizations that will help you to get started is also available in the appendix. Of course, you can always hold your own meeting. Put a notice in the newspaper. Invite a speaker or use what you already know to spark a discussion. Try to schedule regular meetings. Support groups can be very useful places to exchange information on PMS and to express feelings about being a woman. From these groups has come, and will continue to come, much of the impetus to continue investigating the causes and treatments of PMS.

7

GOING TO THE DOCTOR FOR PMS

If you have severe symptoms of PMS that are not relieved by self-help measures, you should seek a gynecologist or general practitioner who can help you. Many physicians are now familiar with the basic theories on the causes and treatments for PMS. Some of the doctors may be found in PMS clinics located in many cities.

Look for a doctor who will take you seriously and let you take an active part in your treatment. You may be told that your complaint is normal and you just have to learn to live with it. Or a doctor may suggest that you have a psychological, not a medical, problem.

Don't get discouraged. Keep in mind that PMS *is* a medical problem and that there *are* treatments available. Make an appointment with another, better-informed doctor, if necessary. Persist until you get effective treatment and help for your symptoms.

DIAGNOSIS

Schedule your first appointment with the gynecologist or general practitioner in your postmenstrual period, not in the two weeks before menstruation. Generally speaking, this is a time when you are in better control of your emotions and can speak more objectively about your symptoms. Also, you are less vulnerable and less apt to accept unsatisfactory suggestions or recommendations.

Try to bring a parent or very close friend along on your first visit to the doctor. The other person can confirm or lend weight to your description of the symptoms. It will show the doctor that you take PMS seriously enough to involve someone else in your efforts to control the disorder. This kind of involvement can also help you strengthen a relationship that may have become difficult and strained during your bouts with PMS.

When you sit down with the doctor, he or she will take your medical history. The first two questions most likely to be asked are: What are your symptoms? When do they appear?

Your menstrual chart for three months (see p. 46) will come in very handy at this time. Be sure that it is clear and easy to read. Make the key to abbreviations legible, and the levels of severity should stand out. Perhaps you can highlight the symptom-free days to make the presentation even better.

The doctor will probably then need some other information on your menstrual history: when menstruation started (approximate date and your age at the time), the length of your cycle (number of days from onset of flow to the next onset of flow), and any special aspects (for example, menstrual irregularities, missed periods, especially heavy or light flow). Most doctors will want to know, too, how your symptoms affect your ability to conduct your daily affairs, the steps you have taken to help yourself, and the results. Be sure to mention other doctors, if any, that you have consulted, their diagnoses, treatments, and outcomes.

While speaking with the doctor, remember that there is no way to test for PMS. The diagnosis depends on the way you relate your experience with PMS—the physical and psychological symptoms. That is why you have to be as clear and well-informed as possible. Since PMS *is not a subject taught in medical school,* be prepared to discuss what you know and have read about PMS. Consider yourself the doctor's partner in the process of making a diagnosis.

Of course, any diagnosis of PMS must include a thorough physical examination. The main purpose is to determine if any of the premenstrual symptoms arise from some underlying disease condition. If not, the doctor may advise treating the purely premenstrual symptoms in a number of different ways, from conservative to more radical.

VITAMIN THERAPY

One of the mildest and simplest treatments some doctors suggest involves taking daily amounts of vitamin B_6, also called pyridoxine. Many consider this treatment the "treatment of first choice."

Vitamin B_6 is naturally present in your body from the foods you eat. But in some people, this is not enough. They suffer a deficiency of vitamin B_6 that cannot be made up by a change in diet alone. Many find that, in addition to eating foods rich in vitamin B_6 (see p. 40), taking supplementary dosages can be very helpful.

There are many theories that try to explain the reason for the common deficiency of B_6 in women with PMS. One idea is that high levels of estrogen deplete the vitamin. The deficiency is associated with depression, bloating, and acne—three typical symptoms of PMS. Also, high levels of B_6 are needed for the proper functioning of the hypothalamus, the control center for the menstrual cycle.

61

The doctor may prescribe daily multivitamin pills that contain between 40 and 100 milligrams of B_6. Taking such amounts will not cause any difficulty because this vitamin is water-soluble; excess amounts will be excreted in the urine.

Occasionally, you may be asked to buy special B_6 tablets that contain as much as 800 milligrams of B_6. At that level, you may very well experience some unpleasant side effects, such as headaches, dizziness, or nausea. A good doctor will either adjust the dosage or advise you to stop taking the vitamin, especially if it does not seem to be helping the condition.

Doctors, you will find, vary in the schedule they advise for taking the vitamin. Dr. Michael G. Brush, for example, has had good results with patients who start the pills a few days before the expected onset of PMS and continue the therapy until a few days after menstruation begins. Dr. Harrison, on the other hand, has found that it is more advantageous to take the vitamin daily throughout the cycle. Listen to your own doctor's suggestion. Then observe how well the dosage and frequency work for you.

When the right dosage is found, most doctors agree, you will notice a sudden improvement. For many women, nine months of vitamin B_6 supplements are all that is necessary to make the symptoms disappear. Others have found that the symptoms return after vitamin therapy ends. These women are often advised to resume taking vitamin B_6 regularly or premenstrually.

The medical literature shows some remarkable results with vitamin B_6 therapy. St. Thomas's Hospital in London reports that over 80 percent of women with premenstrual headaches were cured. About 65 percent of those with premenstrual tension were either cured or helped to feel very much better.

Still, some experts are skeptical. In a review of the literature on PMS, Drs. Reid and Yen of UCLA criticized the vitamin B_6 theory. They advised further clinical trials. A group of doctors reported in *The New England Journal of Medicine* that taking vitamin B_6 in exceedingly large amounts can cause nerve damage.

DIURETICS

Diuretics, you remember, are substances that help remove water from your tissues. Often they are prescribed to reduce the bloating associated with PMS, but they can be dangerous.

While diuretics sometimes help relieve breast swelling and fight weight gain, more often they just create a bigger demand for liquids. What's more, they can tend to make you feel more tired and lethargic. Excessive use of diuretics can upset the levels of potassium and sodium in your body, worsening the symptoms of PMS. Prolonged use of diuretics can be harmful to your health.

PROGESTERONE THERAPY

Progesterone, as you know, is a sex hormone that is crucial in preparing the uterus for pregnancy. Where there is a deficiency of progesterone in your blood or an imbalance of progesterone in relation to estrogen, you may experience the symptoms of PMS.

The idea of raising the level of progesterone in the blood of PMS patients is an old one. Dr. Dalton has been using natural progesterone therapy in England since 1948. In the United States, doctors started to use the hormone in June 1981. Most reports on progesterone therapy have been very good. In Dr. Norris's study of 100 patients with severe symptoms of PMS who received progesterone therapy, he found 77 became free of the symptoms and the rest improved significantly.

If your doctor prescribes progesterone, you will probably take it from the time of ovulation until the start of menstruation. Changes may be made in the schedule. If your symptoms appear with ovulation, the progesterone may be started earlier. If the symptoms last fewer than five days, you may be told to begin taking the progesterone just a few days before the expected onset of PMS. If your menstrual cycle happens to be irregular or the symptoms continue past menstruation, the progesterone may still be stopped at the time of expected onset of your period.

Natural progesterone is not always the preferred treatment because of certain difficulties in administering the hormone. The chief problem is that if it is taken by mouth, it is digested and broken down by the body, doing nothing to correct the hormone imbalance.

Neither of the two methods that are used are particularly convenient. In one method, suppositories containing the hormone are inserted in the rectum or the vagina. The other method is to give the progesterone as an injection, usually in the buttocks.

Suppositories, the more usual form, are difficult to obtain because at this time no drug company is manufacturing them in the United States. The chief sources are certain druggists who prepare them individually. This tends to make them very expensive. Injections, which can be very painful and may cause allergic reactions, are used mostly for women who are hospitalized, suicidal, potentially dangerous to others, or not responsive to suppositories.

Your doctor, with your help, will decide on how big a dose you require. Individual needs vary considerably. Dr. Cynthia W. Cooke of the University of Pennsylvania School of Medicine reportedly starts patients off on 20 milligrams a day. A larger dose, between 200 and 400 milligrams, is prescribed by Dr. Dalton. The upper limit appears to be in the 4,000 to 6,000 milligram range.

Should you be given progesterone, it can take some time to get results. Usually you will start the hormone four or five days before your period and take it until the onset of menstruation. The doctor may advise you to take the hormone for three cycles, or until you have no more complaints. Or you may be told to gradually cut back the amount by starting it a little later each month. If the symptoms return, you may have to resume using the hormone for a while at least.

Although progesterone therapy has been used for nearly forty years, no one knows just why it works. Some physicians believe that progesterone's success is because it is an analgesic (reduces pain) and a sedative (calms and quiets). "Progesterone just makes me feel good," says one sufferer using this treatment.

Many doctors, including Drs. Dalton and Norris, believe that there is little or no danger of cancer with progesterone therapy. A few doctors, however, cite animal studies that suggest progesterone may increase the danger of breast tumors or cancer.

There seems to be a few serious side effects with this treatment. You may notice these changes if you decide to use progesterone. Too much progesterone can make you euphoric, hyperactive, or unable to fall asleep at night. Or, you may get increased menstrual cramps. Progesterone may make it more likely for vaginal infections to occur. Should you develop any of these symptoms, report them promptly to your doctor. He or she will probably cut the amount of progesterone you take, and the discomfort will very likely disappear.

In the United States, progesterone is usually manufactured from soybeans or yams, under the supervision of the Food and Drug Administration (FDA). The FDA allows it to be made for injections, but not in suppository form. As soon as research proves it safe, the manufacture of suppositories will be permitted as well.

While the FDA has approved progesterone for

human use, it has never suggested its use for PMS. In February 1983, though, the FDA gave the go-ahead signal to several large-scale research projects on progesterone. This may be the first step toward eventually recommending the drug for the treatment of PMS.

Some people get confused between natural progesterone and most synthetic progestogens. Synthetic progestogens, such as are found in the contraceptive pill, for example, do not have the same beneficial effect on PMS as progesterone. In fact, they may actually lower the progesterone levels. In most cases this makes the PMS worse because it causes water retention. According to Dr. Dalton, synthetic progestogens can even suppress the body's supply of the natural hormone.

Some drug companies and doctors are promoting progestogens nevertheless. "It's the commercial attitude," says Dr. Dalton. Unfortunately the term *progesterone* is too often used mistakenly to refer to progestogens. Because the two are frequently confused, be sure to find out exactly what you are getting if your doctor prescribes progesterone.

NEW DRUGS

Growing awareness and interest in PMS is speeding up the pace of research. A number of promising new drugs are now being tested. Bromocryptine is prescribed by some doctors who believe it to be effective in relieving the pain of swollen, tender breasts and other symptoms of water retention. But while some experimenters are getting encouraging results, most others find it dangerous. Some researchers working in England have found that users get unpleasant side effects, including nausea and lowered blood pressure.

At the Johns Hopkins University School of Medicine, Dr. Nelson H. Hendler is conducting studies with another experimental drug, spironolactone. In his preliminary report, Dr. Hendler wrote that he was able to rid six out of seven women of hormonal imbalance with three months of spironolactone treatment. Other research, however, has shown that the drug causes malignancies in rats.

A whole group of drugs, known as antiprostaglandins, are now being used to treat PMS. They have been found to provide relief for premenstrual pain believed due to excessive amounts of prostaglandins in the body. Prostaglandins help regulate muscular contractions in the uterus, among other organs of the body.

Antiprostaglandins are taken by mouth before and during the time of the symptoms. Motrin, Ponstel, and Anaprox are some of the more common drugs in this group. One doctor who is studying the use of Ponstel to treat PMS is Dr. Penny Wise Budoff. Dr. Budoff discovered that Ponstel relieved breast pain, bloating and nausea, as well as menstrual pain. But it did not have any effect on the emotional symptoms of PMS. The most common side effects with Ponstel were found to be nausea, and increased amounts of gas and diarrhea.

At the premenstrual clinic in Massachusetts headed by Dr. Ronald V. Norris, menstrual charts, interviews and physical examinations are used to determine whether or not each patient who seeks help has PMS. Some women who do are offered natural progesterone injections or suppositories. Others are helped through group psychotherapy, biofeedback, and hypnosis.

PMS Action, a non-profit organization in Madison, Wisconsin, was formed in 1980 to educate women about PMS. The group has a list of doctors and clinics in the United States where you can go for treatment for PMS. They also provide addresses of places across the country where progesterone therapy is available.

With all the help now at hand, there is no longer any need to suffer the extreme physical or psychological discomforts of PMS.

8

SOCIAL
AND LEGAL
ISSUES

There is little doubt that PMS is a serious problem for many women. If you have severe PMS symptoms, you may find that it disrupts your activities at school or your performance on the job. It can interfere with your personal relationships, cause you to lose your concentration, and make you clumsier and more apt to have accidents. It may limit your success in sports competitions, or in music, dance, or dramatic presentations. PMS has even been linked to criminal activity.

Women are now entering the job market in record numbers. They are preparing themselves for every kind of career—from astronaut to zoo doctor. If the menstrual cycle affects their abilities and capacities, are women stable or reliable enough to hold positions of power within our society? Will PMS become an excuse to keep women out of responsible jobs? Will any mental upset that has nothing to do with a woman's period be explained as "biological inferiority"? Should PMS be accepted as a defense for child abuse, assault, or any other criminal acts?

THE EFFECTS
OF PMS

Recent findings point up some ways that PMS symptoms affect performance. A study of some boarding schools in England revealed that the girls tended to earn most of their poor marks for sloppy work and bad conduct at the premenstrual time of each month. Researchers found a lowering of mental-ability scores on tests taken by women in the British armed services during the premenstrual period.

Nearly half of all absenteeism by working women was found to occur in the days before menstruation. Costs to American industry have been estimated at about 8 percent of all wages paid. In other countries, the costs are comparable: 3 percent in Italy and England, and 5 percent in Sweden. The greatest number of accidents on the job also seem to come in the forty-eight hours before the start of menses. And 50 percent of all emergency hospital admissions in London take place in the premenstrual period.

Tasks that are usually managed easily can become hard to handle when you are suffering the symptoms of PMS. Top students do poorly in their school work; judges and teachers make poor decisions; cooks lose their senses of taste and smell; outstanding athletes are defeated at games and races; beautiful actresses and models get pimples and look puffy.

Some countries recognize the reality of PMS. In Argentina, according to law, women must be allowed time off from work during their premenstrual period. In India, it's the custom for women to be relieved of housework at that time.

The idea that women are periodically unable to function due to menstrual-related problems goes far back in history. In 1890, for example, the French physician Dr. S. Icard wrote that because of "the psychical and physical state of women during the menstrual periods . . . she should not administer public affairs." Recently Dr. Edgar Berman, in a 1970 debate with Dr. Estelle Ramey, said that women were subject to a "raging hormonal imbalance." What's more, he asserted, "It's all evolutionary and genetic." Women are not fit to be presidents of banks, he continued, because they would make bad loans during "that particular period."

But obviously women *are* functioning as bank presidents—and as brain surgeons, pilots, computer specialists, and workers in every difficult, demanding, and dangerous field imaginable. Of course, not all have PMS. But many do. How do they cope?

COPING WITH PMS

Dr. Norris has evaluated about 2,000 women in his PMS clinic to date. About 1,200 have careers outside the home. Almost all say that their PMS has had a bad effect on their work. But most have found various ways to deal with their condition.

One method is to seek improvement by themselves or with the help of a doctor. They adjust their diets, undertake daily exercise, relaxation, and stress-reduction programs, and, if necessary, start on vitamin or progesterone therapy.

They also try to adjust to the situation. Examples of women who are learning to handle PMS in a positive way come from all over the world. One woman who works as an executive in a Chicago business firm says, "Until I found out I had PMS, I was afraid to advance in my firm. For five days of every month I was a wreck. I'd lose my temper and say things I was sorry about. Now, with treatment, I have nothing to fear. I know which situations to avoid—and when."

A woman lawyer in Canada said that she became so forgetful that she couldn't go to court the day or so before her period. Now she arranges her schedule more carefully. She avoids court appearances when she's "not up to them." A Swedish actress who cannot remember her lines or fit into her costumes when she is premenstrual makes arrangements for her understudy to appear for her on those days. The bakery worker who finds that she can't stand on her feet for a few days before the start of her menses asks her employer for flexible hours. A number of short breaks during the day, instead of a single lunch hour, make it far easier for her to get through the premenstrual period.

A nurse who used to work the 10 P.M. to 6 A.M. shift at a California hospital found that night work made her symptoms worse. She asked for a change of shift—and soon was feeling much better. A salesperson at a large department store takes advantage of the lounge that her store provides for the employees. A tennis star plans her important matches away from her menstrual times. Some professional athletes and performers take contraceptive pills to control the dates of their menstrual cycles.

Experts who work with women who have PMS find that many use monthly changes as a source of strength, not weakness. A busy real estate agent schedules all her evictions and demands for late-rent payments "on days when my hormones are raging." A number of artists and writers with PMS believe that they do their most creative work premenstrually. One ceramist describes the feeling as a "monthly surge of energy." At such times, she says, "no task is impossible or too difficult."

PUTTING THE
BLAME ON PMS

Since the symptoms of PMS are real, and can be very disruptive, some think that women with PMS should be given special consideration. Teachers, employers, judges, family members, and friends, they say, should be told when a woman has PMS. It should be taken into account when evaluating the way she acts and what she accomplishes during her premenstrual period.

Many others oppose this view. They hold that using PMS as an excuse for poor performance or behavior will be bad for women—and for society. Alan A. Stone, a psychiatrist and law professor at Harvard University, puts it this way: "I don't see why it is any different than any other illness." Perhaps that is why women with PMS are educating themselves—and others—about PMS. They are putting the various self-help approaches to work for them. And they are seeking medical treatment when they find it is necessary.

In 1979, while working in a pub in England, thirty-year-old Sandy Smith stabbed a barmaid three times through the heart, killing her instantly. On the basis of a diagnosis of PMS made by Dr. Dalton, the court reduced the charge from murder to manslaughter. The judge then sentenced Smith to three years probation, provided that she continue progesterone treatment.

The following year, also in England, thirty-seven-year-old Christine English, after a fight with her boy friend, ran him down with a car, pinning him to a light pole. As a result of his injuries, he died a few days later. Because she had a history of PMS, the charge was changed from murder to manslaughter. The woman was placed on probation, provided that she did not drive and was willing to accept treatment for her PMS.

In Brooklyn, New York, in 1982, Shirley Santos, age twenty-five, was accused of beating her four-year-old daughter severely. Santos's lawyer announced that she would base her defense on the fact that her client had PMS, since the attack coincided with the onset of her period. The case, however, was settled out of court, with the judge freeing Ms. Santos after she agreed to stay in a counseling program for one year.

In these three cases, women used PMS as part of their legal defense against criminal charges. Do you believe that women who commit crimes during the premenstrual time should be freed of responsibility for their deeds? Or do you feel that PMS is no excuse for antisocial behavior? Opinions are sharply divided on this issue. In fact, PMS is emerging as one of the very important controversies of our time.

Those who view PMS as a disabling "disease" cite various studies to bolster their claim. For example, of 132 women treated at the Premenstrual Syndrome Clinic, University College Hospital, London, in 1977, 37 percent had been admitted to a mental hospital at least once, 34 percent had attempted either suicide or homicide, 9 percent had periods of alcoholism, 6 percent had been accused of some crime, and 6 percent had a history of child battering. An international survey of women in prison showed that over half committed their crimes just before or immediately after menstruation.

As long ago as 1854, Martha Brixey was acquitted of murder on the grounds of temporary insanity caused by "obstructed menstruation." The legal code in Great Britain accepts PMS as a mitigating factor in the sentences of women found guilty of violent crimes, even though it cannot be used as a legal defense. In France, PMS is considered part of a temporary-insanity plea.

PMS has not yet been tested as a defense in American courts. In the Shirley Santos assault case, her attorney, Stephanie Benson, argued that the cause of her client's violent behavior was PMS. When describing the child beating, Santos said, "I didn't mean to hurt her; I just got my period." Attorney Benson held that the mother had blacked out, or suffered spontaneous hypoglycemia, which sometimes accompanies PMS. Hypoglycemia, the abnormally low level of sugar in the blood, has already been used as a legal defense in cases of murder and assault. It is known to cause aggression, violent outbursts, amnesia, and fatigue—all symptoms that were present in the Santos case.

Objectors to Stephanie Benson's use of the PMS defense were very widespread. Among them was Sybil Shainwald, of the National Women's Health Network, who said that she is "unalterably opposed to PMS as a defense."

The District Attorney in the Shirley Santos case, Elizabeth Holtzman, asserted that there was no evidence of PMS. A defense plea on these grounds, she said, would discredit all women. "I think that we ought to be able to say that women can be held accountable for their acts just as men are." Her office had examined 3,000 medical journals, but they could not find anything indicating that women lose complete control over their emotions during the premenstrual period. Nothing showed that women with PMS are unable to tell right from wrong. She warned that acceptance of PMS as a disabling condition would tend to influence unfavorably women's position in divorce proceedings and custody battles. It might even justify the physical violence perpetrated against so many women.

We all know that women with PMS are not the only ones to undergo mood swings and changes in efficiency. Some scientists point to the cyclical patterns of physical, emotional, and behavioral change brought about by hormonal factors in men as well as in women. A study in Denmark found that men have a monthly cycle of production of testosterone, the male sex hormone. Research in Japan uncovered evidence that men's cycles affected their efficiency at work, ability to make sound decisions, and chances of being involved in an accident. Yet no one is considering using the male hormonal cycle as a defense plea.

Dr. Franz Halberg has collected data showing that

men go through cyclical changes in strength of grip and beard growth. Another researcher, Dr. Gideon Seaman, believes that the male monthly cycle may be even more of a problem than the female cycle. That is because it is not associated with a concrete, observable event, such as the onset of menstruation.

If cycles of hormonal change are universal, and if such changes are linked to criminal behavior, then hormonal imbalance may become a common criminal plea. It may turn out, according to one theory, that every criminal is chemically disturbed in some way. But since approximately 90 percent of all violent crimes are committed by men, this hormone imbalance is probably not an important factor in violent behavior, after all.

Before PMS can become a defense plea, it would seem, several points would have to be clarified. For instance, we have to have an exact definition of PMS, as well as an objective medical test for the condition. Scientists do not yet know in what way or ways women who experience PMS differ from those who do not. No one is able to draw a line separating the moderate sufferers from those with severe conditions, which Dr. Dalton and others believe may cause violent and criminal behavior.

THE LAST WORD

Menstruation and the premenstrual syndrome are no longer subjects to be whispered about or regarded with shame and embarrassment. Now is the time to bring PMS out into the open. Girls and boys, women and men, doctors and lawyers—everyone must be educated to the fact that PMS is a medical condition with real physical and psychological symptoms. It is a subject that needs to be discussed and debated as openly as any other painful or difficult condition of human life.

Carefully planned large-scale research is still sorely lacking. We need a better understanding of PMS. We have to find new and improved ways to treat it. And we must search for answers to the many legal and moral questions raised by PMS. The results will help women become truly free to shape their own destinies.

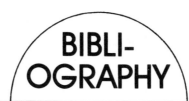

BIBLIOGRAPHY

Bender, Stephanie and Kathleen Kelleher. *PMS: A Positive Program to Gain Control.* Los Angeles: The Body Press, 1986.

Bender, Stephanie DeGraff. *PMS: Questions and Answers.* Los Angeles: The Body Press, 1989.

Budoff, Penny Wise. *No More Menstrual Cramps and Other Good News.* New York: Penguin, 1981.

Dalton, Katharina. *The Premenstrual Syndrome and Progesterone Therapy.* Chicago: Year Book Medical Publishers, 1985.

Dalton, Katharina. *Once A Month.* Fourth, revised edition. Claremont, CA: Hunter House, 1990.

Delaney, Janice, Mary Jane Lupton, and Emily Toth. *The Curse.* New York: Dutton, 1976.

Eagen, Andrea Boroft. *Why am I So Miserable If These Are the Best Years of My Life?* Philadelphia: Lippincott, 1976.

Halas, Celia. *Relief from Premenstrual Syndrome.* New York: Frederick Fell Publishers, 1984.

Harrison, Michelle. *Self Help for Premenstrual Syndrome.* New and expanded edition. New York: Random House, 1985.

Kass-Annese, Barbara and Hal Danzer. *A Complete Guide to the Treatment of Premenstrual Syndrome.* Santa Monica, CA: Patterns Publishing, 1984.

Lanson, Lucienne. *From Woman to Woman.* New York: Knopf, 1981.

Lark, Susan. *Premenstrual Syndrome Self Help Book.* New York: Forman Publishing, Inc., 1984.

Lauersen, Niels and Eileen Stukane. *Listen to Your Body.* New York: Simon & Schuster, 1982.

Lauersen, Niels H. and Eileen Stukane. *Premenstrual Syndrome and You.* New York: Pinnacle Books, Inc., 1983.

Norris, Ronald V. with Colleen Sullivan. *PMS: Premenstrual Syndrome.* New York: Rawson, 1983.

Seaman, Barbara. *Women and the Crisis in Sex Hormones.* New York: Rawson, 1977.

Witt, Reni L. *PMS: What Every Woman Should Know About Premenstrual Syndrome.* New York: Stein & Day, 1983.

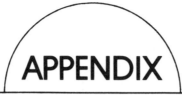

APPENDIX

SELECTED SOURCES OF INFORMATION AND HELP

Endometriosis Association
585 N. 76th Place
Milwaukee, WI 53223
(1-800) 992-3636
(414) 962-8972

HEALTH-PAC (Health Policy Advisory Committee)
17 Murray Street
New York, NY 10007
(212) 267-8890

Publications on women's health among other topics.

Health Research Group
2000 P Street, NW
Washington D.C. 20036
(202) 872-0320

National Health Information Center
P.O. Box 1133
Washington D.C. 20013-1133
(1-800) 336-4797
(301) 565-4167

National Self-Help Clearinghouse
Graduate School and University Center
City University of New York
33 West 42nd Street, Room 1227
New York, NY 10036
(212) 840-7606

Publishes manuals on self-help groups

National Women's Health Network
1325 G Street, NW
Lower Level B
Washington D.C. 20005
(202) 347-1140

General information on women's health issues.
Refers to local health groups.

For a listing of referral sources or groups in the USA, consult Dr. Katharina Dalton's *Once A Month*, Fourth Edition, 1990 (see the order form at the back of this book), or send a self-addressed stamped envelope to the publisher asking for a PMS Clinics and Support Groups List. There is no charge for this service.

INDEX

Aches and pains, 22–23
Alcoholism, 32–33
Amenorrhea, 12
Antiprostaglandins, 67
Asthma, 23

Binge eating, 33
Biography, 79–80
Bleeding, 9
    cause of heavy, 11
Bloating, 20–21
Blood sugar, low, 39–40
Breast tenderness and
    swelling, 19–20
Bromocryptine, 66
Bruising, 25–26
Brush, Michael, 19, 37, 62

Causes of PMS, 35–44
Chart, keeping of, 45–48

Clinical depression, 31
Clumsiness and poor
    coordination, 25
Conception, 9
Congestive dysmenor-
    rhea, 22–23
Conjunctivitis, 24
Constipation, 21
Coordination, poor, 25
Coping with PMS, 71–72
Cramps, 12–13

Daily report, 48, 50
Dalton, Katharina, 2, 5–6,
    12, 13, 18, 19, 23, 24,
    31, 35–38
Depression, 30–31
Diagnosis, 59–61
Diuretics, 63
Dizziness, 26

Doctors' visits, 59–68
Drugs, new, 66–67

Eating habits, 50–52
    eating binges, 33
    food cravings, 33–34
    foods to avoid, 52–54
Effects of PMS, 70–71
Epilepsy, 23–24
Estrogen, 8, 22, 35, 37, 61
Exercise and relaxation
    techniques, 55–56
Eye problems, 24

Fainting, 25–26
Fallopian tubes, 9
"Flight or flee" syndrome,
    40
Follicular phase of men-
    strual cycle, 8
Food cravings, 33–34
Frank, Robert, 4
FSH (Follicle Stimulating
    Hormone), 8

Glaucoma, 24

Harrison, Dr., 62
Haskell, Roger, 4
Headaches, 18–19
Hormonal problems, 35–
    38
Hypothalamus, 8, 9, 12,
    61

Irritability, 29–30

Lanson, Lucienne, 21
Legal defense and PMS,
    72–76
LH (Luteinizing Hor-
    mone), 8, 9
Low blood sugar, 39–40
Luteal phase, 9

Mattson, Richard, 23
Menarche, 7
Menopause, 7
Menstrual cycle, 7–16
    follicular phase of, 8
Menstrual difficulties, 11–13
Menstruation, 7, 8–11
Migraine headache, 19

Neurotransmitters, 43
Norris, Ronald, 30, 33,
    56, 67, 71
Nose and throat ailments,
    24–25

Organizations, 81–82

Pink eye, 24
Pituitary gland, 12
PMS
    causes of, 35–44
    coping with, 71–72
    diagnosis, 59–61
    effects of, 70–71
    legal defense and,
        72–76
    problem of, 4–5
    symptoms, 5, 17–34

PMS (*continued*)
   what it is, 2–3
   what it is not, 3–4
PMS Action, 67
Problem of PMS, 4–5
Progesterone, 9, 11, 35
   therapy, 63–66
Prolactin, 37
Prostaglandins, 13, 67
Psychological symptoms,
   27–34
Puberty, 7
Pyridoxine, 40, 61

Radioimmunoassay, 37
Relaxation techniques,
   55–56
Remedy, 5–6

Self-help, 14–15, 45–58
Sinus headache, 18
Skin disorders, 21–22
Smell, loss of, 25
Social and legal issues,
   69–78

Spasmodic dysmenorrhea,
   12–13, 14, 22–23
Spironolactone, 66–67
Stress, effect on men-
   strual cycle, 11–12
   managing, 56–58
Suicide, 31
Swelling, breast, 19–20
Symptoms of PMS, 5, 17–34

Talking it out, 58
Taylor, R.W., 37
Tension, 28–29
Tension headache, 18–19
Throat ailments, 24–25
Tiredness, 31–32

Vacuum headache, 18
Vitamin B6, 61–62
Vitamin deficiency, 40–41
Vitamin therapy, 61–63

Water retention, 38–39
Weight gain and bloating,
   20–21

Hunter House
HEALTH & FAMILY BOOKS

THE NEW A-TO-Z OF WOMEN'S HEALTH: A Concise Encyclopedia   by Christine Ammer
> Over 1000 expert, informative entries covering birth to old age. Featuring charts, diagrams and an important appendix of resources, this book is an essential reference for women of all ages.
> *Soft Cover ... 496 pages ... $16.95*

FEELING GREAT: A Guide to Natural Highs
by Nancy Levinson and Joanne Rocklin, Ph.D.
> Being high is a natural, healthy state—and we don't need drugs to get there. This vitally important book provides ideas, resources, and guidelines that are easily overlooked in society, especially today.
> *Soft Cover ... 112 pages ... 2nd Edition ... $7.95*

MENOPAUSE WITHOUT MEDICINE   by Linda Ojeda, Ph.D.
> Preparing for a healthy menopause can never begin too early. Ojeda's natural approach focuses on nutrition, physical conditioning, beauty care, and psychological health. This completely updated edition contains the latest medical information.
> *Soft Cover ... 304 pages ... 2nd Edition ... Illustrated ...$12.95*

ONCE A MONTH: The *Original* Premenstrual Syndrome Handbook   by Katharina Dalton, M.D.
> The first book—and still the best—to explain clearly the symptoms, effects and complete treatment of Premenstrual Syndrome. By the acknowledged pioneer in the field.
> *Soft Cover ... 272 pages ... Illustrated ... 4th Edition ... $9.95*

SELF-HELP FOR PMS   by Michelle Harrison, M.D.
> Symptoms, causes and treatments for PMS, with emphasis on self-help, including diet, exercise, vitamins, progesterone, psychotherapy, and more.
> *Soft cover ... 192 pages ... 2nd Edition ... $9.95*

SEXUAL HEALING: A Self-Help Program to Enhance Your Sensuality and Overcome Common Sexual Problems
by Barbara Keesling, Ph.D.
> Exercises allow the reader to evaluate his or her sexual needs and develop a program to share with a partner. Also teaches specific skills for relaxing, reducing anxiety, and maximizing sexual enjoyment.
> *Soft cover ... 288 pages ... $12.95*

Prices subject to change without notice
See over for ordering and discounts

ORDER FORM

NAME

ADDRESS

CITY/STATE   ZIP

COUNTRY (outside USA)   POSTAL CODE

TITLE	QTY	PRICE	TOTAL
The New A-to-Z of Women's Health	| @	$ 16.95	
Feeling Great	| @	$ 7.95	
Menopause Without Medicine *2nd Edition*	| @	$ 12.95	
Once A Month *4th Edition*	| @	$ 9.95	
PMS: Premenstrual Syndrome *3rd Edition*	| @	$ 7.95	
Self-Help for PMS	| @	$ 9.95	
Sexual Healing	| @	$ 12.95	

Shipping costs:
First book: $2.00
($3.00 for Canada)
Each additional book:
$.50 ($1.00 for
Canada)
For UPS rates and
bulk orders call us at
(510) 865-5282

TOTAL	
Less discount @_____%	(_____)
TOTAL COST OF BOOKS	
Calif. residents add sales tax	
Shipping & handling	
TOTAL ENCLOSED	
Please pay in U.S. funds only	

❑ Check   ❑ Money Order   ❑ Visa   ❑ M/C

Card # _____ Exp date _____

Signature _____

Complete and mail to:

Hunter House Inc., Publishers
2200 Central Ave. Ste. 202, Alameda CA 94501
Phone (510) 865-5282 Fax (510) 865-4295

❑ Check here to receive our book catalog